Dr Dawn's
health
check

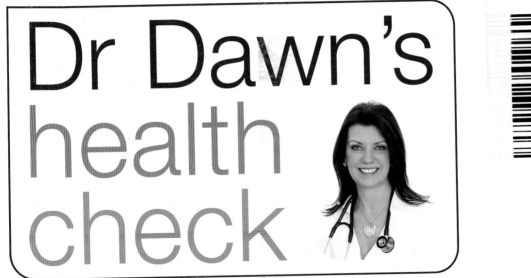

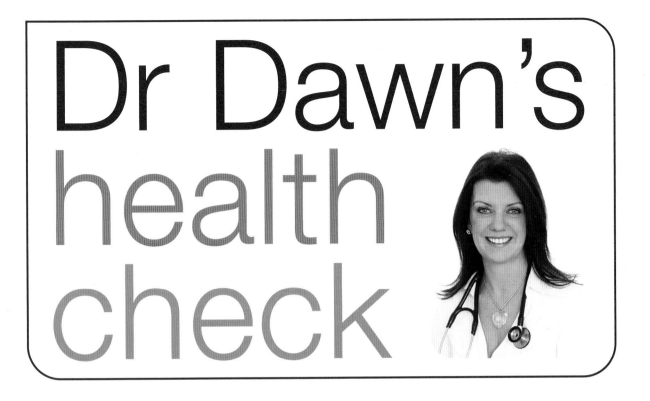

Dr Dawn's
health
check

MITCHELL BEAZLEY

Dr Dawn's health check
Dawn Harper

First published in Great Britain in 2007 by Mitchell Beazley,
an imprint of Octopus Publishing Group Limited,
2–4 Heron Quays, London E14 4JP.
© Octopus Publishing Group Limited 2007
Text © Dawn Harper 2007

A CIP catalogue record for this book is available from the
British Library.

ISBN 13: 978 1 84533 309 6
ISBN 10: 1 845533 309 8

While the medical advice contained in this edition is as accurate
and comprehensive as possible it is only intended as general
advice, and should not be used as a substitute for the advice that
you receive from your own doctor. You are advised to consult your
doctor for specific information concerning your health.

The publisher, editors or author cannot accept responsibility for
any consequences arising from the use thereof or from the
information contained therein.

Commissioning Editors: Anna Sanderson, Hannah Barnes-Murphy
Designer: Gaelle Lochner
Senior Designer: Juliette Norsworthy
Editorial Consultant: Daphne Razazan
Senior Editor: Hannah McEwen
Medical Editors: Jemima Dunne, Martyn Page
Proofreader: Alyson Silverwood
Photography: Ruth Jenkinson
Production: Peter Hunt
Index: Hilary Bird

Printed and bound by Artes Gráficas Toledo in Spain
Typeset in HelveticaNeue

contents

contents

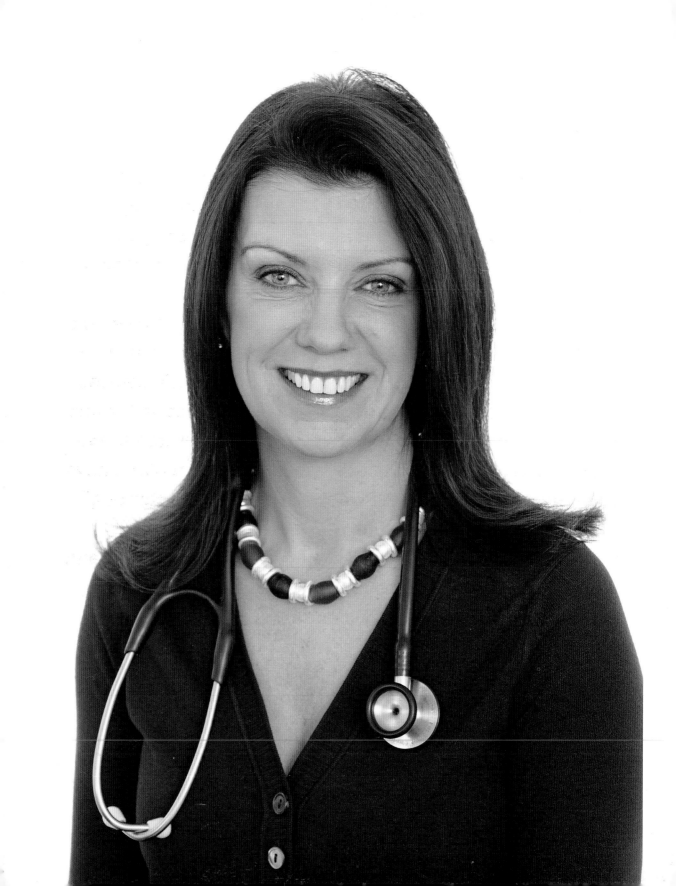

When I was at school my teachers tried hard to persuade me that I was a linguist, and that I should study languages at university. I, on the other hand, like every teenage girl, knew better. From the age of 12 I was adamant that I wanted to be a doctor.

Today I spend half my working week practising medicine, and the other half writing for the press, or talking on television or radio about medical issues. A lot of my writing work involves answering reader's letters and much of the inspiration for this book has come from all those of you who have written to me over the years. So many of my letters begin with "I didn't have the time to ask but," "I didn't want to bother my doctor but," or "it probably sounds silly but."

My hope is that this book will answer all those questions, and the ones you never had time to ask. And it is also something of an apology to Miss Chapman and Mrs Fox who tried so hard all those years ago to get me to study languages – perhaps you were right after all... or maybe we all were!

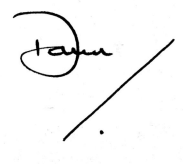

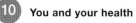

YOU AND YOUR HEALTH

My aim with this book is to help you to help yourself, to know when you need to seek medical advice, and how to make the most of your appointment with your doctor. In many ways, our National Health Service is the envy of the rest of the world, but it also faces many challenges. Understanding your health, and the health of your family, is an important step towards making health services work best for you.

WHO TO ASK FOR ADVICE

There are so many different health services available to people now, that it is hard to know where to turn to for advice – with choice comes confusion. Every week I see patients armed with reams of paper printed from the internet with information that has scared the living daylights out of them.

Throughout the book I have tried to point you in the direction of useful websites that will give you reliable advice, and there is also a 'useful contacts' list at the back for you to refer to. At times I also advise asking your pharmacist – they are highly trained professionals

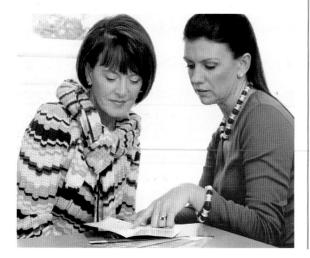

with a wealth of information, and as more drugs become available over the counter, their role in looking after your health may increase. Most pharmacists now have a private area where you can discuss personal matters with your pharmacist.

MAKING AN APPOINTMENT AT YOUR SURGERY

If you need to visit your surgery then there are different people that you can see. If you only need a repeat prescription, you may be able to request this with a telephone call. Some doctors are happy to issue repeat prescriptions over the phone, and your surgery will be able to advise you of their particular procedure.

Most surgeries will offer appointments with a practice nurse, and the practice nurse will be able to deal with many health issues. You may also find that you will be able to get an appointment with the practice nurse sooner than you can with a doctor.

If you are unsure whether you need to see a nurse or doctor, the receptionist will be able to advise. People worry about giving personal details to the receptionist, but you don't have to go into detail, "I have a sore throat," or "it's women's trouble," may be

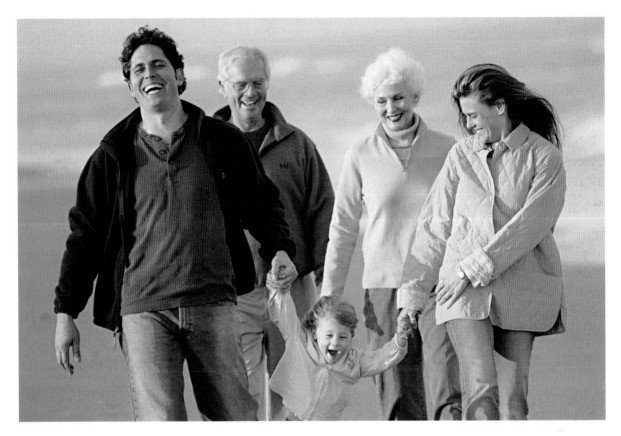

all you need to say. The receptionist is bound by the same rules of confidentiality as the medical staff, and will know the expertise of the doctors and nurses in the practice, so is well equipped to make sure you see the best person. If there is a doctor in your surgery with a particular interest connected to your ailment, the receptionist will be able to let you know.

Make the most of an appointment by being clear in your mind about your concerns, and the information that you need. You could make a list and show it to your doctor – the symptoms may be linked, and if they are not he or she will be able to deal with the most urgent problem first. If you are terrified you have cancer, say so. It may be so obvious to your doctor that you don't that he or she won't even mention it, and you will leave without feeling reassured.

If you have a complicated complaint that will need more time, ask to book a double appointment, and consider taking a friend along with you. Most of us only retain about 20 per cent of the information we receive in a consultation, and your friend may be able to take notes for you to look over later.

GOING TO HOSPITAL

It is best to restrict visits to an accident and emergency department in a hospital for serious problems that you don't know how to deal with. Be aware that depending on the hospital and time you visit, you may be in for a long wait if it is a non-emergency.

You can also dial 999 for serious emergencies, and this book will flag-up some of the occasions when it is necessary to dial 999.

• Our eyes make several hundred tiny movements called saccades every minute • We blink over 16,000 times each day • No two ears are identical • Only our ears and our noses continue to grow throughout our lives • The human noses can differentiate between 10,000 different smells • The number of taste buds in our mouths is usually between 2,000 and 5,000 but there is such huge variation from person to person, it can be as few as 500 or as many as 20,000 • Salivary glands produce over half a litre of saliva every day.

1

Eyes, ears, nose & mouth

Introduction Our faces are what identify us, they reflect our personality, and, if we let them, they allow those around us to see how we feel. The human face is made up of 14 bones, 32 teeth, and over 50 muscles. Facial muscles are different to any other muscles in the body because many of them attach to each other or to skin, rather than to bones. A tiny movement in these muscles can alter the contours of the face to create hundreds of expressions.

The fascinating thing about facial expressions is that they are not specific to culture, gender, or ethnicity – we are all able to recognize a happy, angry or confused face. Our eyebrows go up when we are surprised, our foreheads wrinkle when we are perplexed, and our lips curve up into a smile when we are happy. We normally make these facial expressions without any conscious thought as an immediate response to the emotion that we are experiencing, but we can suppress these expressions if we really concentrate.

Eyes

STYES

These are painful red lumps that form at the base of an eyelash. They may heal of their own accord, or they can become infected.

WHAT YOU CAN DO
In the early stage, bathing the affected area in warm salt water can speed the healing process. If a stye develops a point or discharges pus, check with your doctor as you may need antibiotics.

IF A CYST REMAINS?
Occasionally, a small cyst (called a meibomian cyst) persists after the infection has cleared. If this happens, seek medical advice. I have a low threshold for referring patients with a cyst to an eye specialist to have it removed, as they often become reinfected.

▼ A typical stye causing a painful red lump.

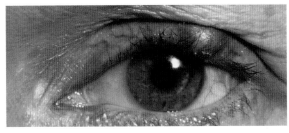

? DID YOU KNOW
What causes bags under the eyes?
Bags under your eyes are rarely a reflection of how much water you drink; it has more to do with age and genetics. As you age, your eyeballs sink into their sockets, squeezing the fat behind the eye into the area below. This, combined with the fact that skin becomes less elastic with age, can cause the bags. Remember that smoking and sun exposure will also exaggerate the whole process.

CONJUNCTIVITIS

This term simply means inflammation of the conjunctiva (the thin covering over the white part of the eye), causing a reddened, itchy eye. Conjunctivitis is common in children, and is likely to get your child sent home from nursery or school faster than almost anything else because it is often contagious.

WHAT CAUSES IT?
Conjunctivitis can be caused by infection, but irritation from chemicals or allergy (to pollens, for example) can also be to blame. The clue is in the discharge from the eye: if there is a clear, watery discharge, it's more likely to be due to allergy or a viral infection (which won't respond to antibiotics); while a thicker, yellow or green discharge means it's probably bacterial and will need antibiotic drops or ointment. Viral and bacterial conjunctivitis are both infectious, but you are not able to catch allergic conjunctivitis from anyone.

WHAT YOU CAN DO
Seek medical advice; bacterial conjunctivitis is highly contagious. I have a low threshold for prescribing drops for both eyes, even if only one is infected – no matter how careful you are, it is easy to rub the infected eye and pass the infection from one eye to the other. If one member of your family has conjunctivitis, you need to ensure that he or she uses separate flannels and towels. Antibiotic ointments may be more practical for very young children, who tend to blink when drops are applied, causing most of the drops to run down their face.

▼ Sore red eyes caused by conjunctivitis.

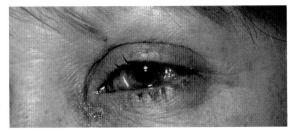

SHORTSIGHTEDNESS

This condition, known as myopia, occurs when the eyeball is too long from front to back, causing a mismatch between the length of the eye, and the focusing power of the cornea (the clear dome in front of the pupil) and the lens at the back of the eye. Although shortsighted people can see close objects, distant ones appear blurred.

WHO IS AFFECTED?

Shortsightedness usually develops in childhood when the eyeball is growing and although it may worsen during the teen years, it tends to stabilize in adulthood.

CAN WATCHING TV MAKE IT WORSE?

There have been concerns about a possible link between the development of myopia and prolonged periods spent doing close-up work or sitting too close to the television, but this hasn't been proven. I take a pragmatic view. I have never stopped my children reading and writing, but I do make them sit away from the TV… and limit their viewing hours! However, all children should have regular eye tests, and especially if there is a history of shortsightedness in the family.

WHAT ARE THE OPTIONS FOR TREATING SHORTSIGHTEDNESS?

Shortsighted people need to wear glasses or contact lenses with a concave lens to correct their vision. Which you choose is a matter of personal preference.

The use of laser surgery to correct shortsightedness has become increasingly popular. A small flap is made in the cornea and a tiny piece of tissue is removed using a laser. The procedure takes about 15 minutes and is done in an outpatient clinic. However, it's expensive, it's a relatively new procedure, and we don't yet know about long-term safety. It's worth noting, too, that laser surgery doesn't stop the normal ageing process of the eye. So people treated for shortsightedness may still need glasses for longsightedness when they are over the age of about 40.

LONGSIGHTEDNESS

This condition, known as hypermetropia, occurs when the eyeball is too short. Long-sighted people find focusing on objects far away easy, but they struggle to see close-up work clearly. This condition tends to start later in life and worsens with age.

CORRECTING THE PROBLEM

Longsightedness can be corrected with glasses or contact lenses with a convex lens. Some people only need them for close work, others need to wear them all the time. Having an eye test every couple of years will pick up the signs early – don't wait until you find yourself holding the newspaper at arm's length in order to be able to read it before you go for an eye test.

▼ Regular eye tests are essential for everyone to identify vision problems as early as possible.

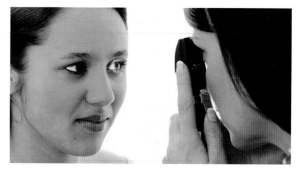

DR DAWN'S HEALTH CHECK
Regular eye tests are essential for all

It's important to pick up vision problems as soon as possible. Eye tests are free for all children under 16 and for those under 19 in full-time education.

• All children under 16 should have their eyes tested every year, especially if eye problems run in the family.

• Adults without any vision problems should be tested every two years, or annually if over 40.

• Adults with vision problems may need more frequent tests; your optometrist can give you advice.

GLAUCOMA

This is a condition caused by raised pressure in the eye, which can damage the optic nerve, causing permanent impairment of vision. Around half a million people in the UK suffer from glaucoma. It accounts for about ten per cent of all new blind registrations. This is a frightening statistic; the good news is that it can be prevented by early detection (by regular eye tests) and treatment.

WHAT ARE THE SYMPTOMS?

If the eye pressure rises quickly (acute glaucoma), it can give you a very painful, red eye – something that is more common in longsighted people and should always be checked out urgently by a doctor. But in the vast majority of cases, the pressure rises slowly (chronic, or long-term, glaucoma) and there are no symptoms.

WHAT YOU CAN DO

The only certain way of knowing if you have glaucoma is to have a full eye test. If you have a family history of glaucoma, you are up to six times more likely to develop it, and you are entitled to free eye tests – so make that appointment. Other groups at increased risk of developing glaucoma include anyone over the age of 40, those with diabetes, people who are shortsighted, and Afro-Caribbeans. If you are in any of these groups, you should get your eyes tested annually.

TREATMENT

A painful, red eye accompanied by haloes appearing around lights is a medical emergency and medical advice should be sought immediately. If the pressure build-up isn't relieved it, can lead to irreversible blindness, but early treatment can help prevent severe damage. Chronic glaucoma can be treated with drops, tablets, or laser surgery. You may need to continue using drops even after surgery, although probably at a lower dose.

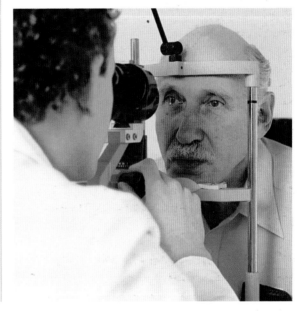

▾ *Early detection of glaucoma by regular eye testing is essential to prevent irreversible blindness.*

🗑 MYTH BUSTERS
Let's take a look at some of the myths that we hear about eyes.

PEOPLE WORKING WITH COMPUTERS BLINK LESS OFTEN	TRUE	This also makes them prone to dry eyes. If you are working in front of a screen for long periods of time, take regular breaks.
COLOUR BLINDNESS ONLY AFFECTS MEN	FALSE	Colour blindness affects both men and women, although it is a genetic condition that is more common in men.
CARROTS CAN HELP YOU SEE IN THE DARK	TRUE	Well, almost! Although carrots will not give you super night vision, they are rich in vitamin A, which helps to maintain healthy eyes.

Ears

TINNITUS

Up to one in five people suffer from tinnitus, a condition that causes a constant noise in one or both ears. People often describe the noise they hear as a buzzing or whooshing, which tends to be worse at night. For most people tinnitus is simply an irritation, but for one in 200 it is so severe that it prevents them from getting on with normal life.

WHAT CAUSES TINNITUS?

It is hard to predict the course of the condition but some things, including stress, tiredness, loud noises, and alcohol, often make symptoms worse. There is very rarely anything sinister causing it.

WHAT YOU CAN DO

Above all, keeping a positive attitude really helps, as do simple masking techniques such as playing a radio or TV in the background or leaving a clock radio on at night. Tinnitus can accompany deafness, in which case wearing a hearing aid will reduce the symptoms. Tinnitus retraining is an option for anyone who feels their symptoms are getting them down, and involves counselling with an in-the-ear sound generator. This takes several months but can make a real difference.

> **! SEEK MEDICAL ADVICE NOW**
> **If you have:**
> - One-sided tinnitus.
> - A sudden onset associated with hearing loss.
> - Dizziness associated with the tinnitus.

FIND OUT MORE
www.tinnitus.org.uk

EARWAX

A build-up of wax in the ear is common and becomes more so with age. Excess earwax affects about one in three people over the age of 50. It can make the ears feel full and, if the wax blocks the ear canal, it can cause deafness.

WHAT CAUSES EARWAX?

Earwax is made up of dead cells and a substance called cerumen, produced by the glands that line the ear canal. The wax traps dirt and protects your eardrum. Some people are more prone to it than others; it affects men more than women.

WHAT YOU CAN DO

Don't try to remove wax with cotton buds as it makes the problem worse. First, try softening the wax with drops that you can get from your chemist. Follow the instructions on the bottle and use them for five days. This is often enough to deal with the problem. If this does not work, make an appointment with the nurse at your doctor's surgery, who can remove the wax by syringing. The drops you applied will have softened the wax, which makes syringing safer – if earwax is impacted, higher pressure is required, which can damage the eardrum. If syringing still doesn't get rid of the wax, then your doctor can refer you to an ear, nose, and throat (ENT) specialist, who will remove it with suction or forceps.

▼ Tilting your head to the side when applying ear drops allows them to work down into the ear canal to soften the wax.

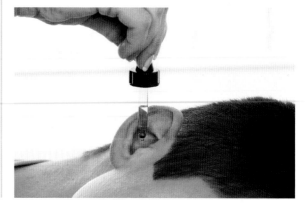

Nose

SINUSITIS

This is inflammation of the lining of the sinuses (air-filled spaces in the skull around the nose) causing facial pain due to a build-up of mucus.

WHAT YOU CAN DO

Around one in 200 common colds develops into sinusitis and if you are prone to it, it's worth trying a good old-fashioned steam inhalation with menthol, morning and evening, at the first sign of any symptoms. This helps liquefy any mucus, making it easier for it to drain from the sinuses and therefore less likely to become infected.

DO DECONGESTANTS HELP?

I am often asked about the role of decongestants for clearing blocked sinuses. Some people certainly find them useful but they must be used short term only. Using them for more than a few days at a time can result in increased congestion when you stop using them.

ARE THERE ANY OTHER TREATMENTS?

Contrary to popular belief, most cases don't require treatment with antibiotics. In fact, according to research, up to two-thirds of patients with sinusitis recover just as quickly without antibiotics as they would if they had them. I tend to reserve using antibiotics for people with systemic symptoms – those with fever and general malaise, as well as the classic facial pain and discharge.

NOSEBLEEDS

Nosebleeds are more common in children. As many as one in 11 children has frequent attacks, but most grow out of them by the time they are 14, and they are rarely anything to worry about.

WHAT CAUSES NOSEBLEEDS?

Although there is often no easily identifiable cause for nosebleeds in children, inflammation and nose-picking make the problem worse. However, nosebleeds that are associated with easy bruising or bleeding elsewhere could indicate an underlying problem. Spontaneous nosebleeds in adults can occasionally be caused by high blood pressure – if you suddenly start getting them, make sure you get your blood pressure checked.

WHAT YOU CAN DO

Lean forward and apply direct pressure to the fleshy part of the nose, pinching it just below the bridge. Do this for ten minutes (timing yourself) and don't be tempted to release the pressure earlier. Tell him or her to spit out any blood that flows into the mouth. After ten minutes, release the pressure; if the bleeding has not stopped, reapply for another ten minutes. If it still hasn't stopped, you will need to go to the nearest hospital accident and emergency department, where the nose can be packed with a special ribbon. Children suffering recurrent attacks should see their doctor.

▼ Pinch the nose just below the bridge to treat a nosebleed.

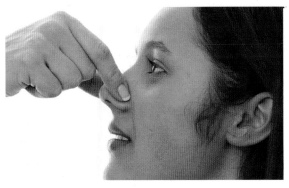

Mouth

COLD SORES

These are small blister-like sores that develop around the mouth, and are caused by a herpes virus. Once you have had the virus, you have it always; it lies dormant in nerve endings and can flare up at any time.

WHAT CAUSES THEM?

Many people get cold sores when they are run down – often if they are feeling stressed or have been ill. Ultraviolet light can also trigger cold sores, which is why so many people develop them when they go on that hard-earned sunshine holiday after a really stressful time.

WHAT YOU CAN DO

Antiviral creams, such as aciclovir (which is available over the counter from your chemist), can shorten the duration of an attack, especially if it is applied as soon as the tell-tale tingling occurs. If you do get cold sores, always keep some at home. Using lipsalve every day (preferably one with a sun-protection factor) may help prevent cold sores. Taking lysine supplements may help reduce the frequency of attacks.

▼ In the early stages, a cold sore looks like a small red blister.

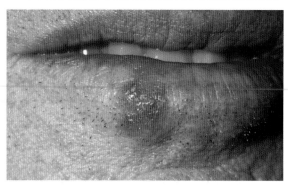

MOUTH ULCERS

One in five of us gets mouth ulcers; they are very common. They usually clear up on their own within a couple of weeks, and like most common conditions there are old wives' tales associated with them. I remember being told that a mouth ulcer was a sign I had been telling lies and perhaps there is some truth in that – stress is a common trigger. I was also told to put salt on the ulcer to stop it hurting – it really stings at first but does help, and warm saline mouthwashes are still used to relieve the pain.

WHEN SHOULD YOU GET MEDICAL ADVICE?

In the vast majority of cases, mouth ulcers can, and should, be treated at home. However, if you have an ulcer that lasts more than three weeks, you should see your doctor or dentist to rule out the possibility of cancer. Anyone who suffers from repeated episodes of mouth ulcers should see their doctor to rule out anaemia or any other conditions associated with them, such as inflammatory bowel disease.

DR DAWN'S HEALTH CHECK
Help with mouth ulcers

You can't cure mouth ulcers, but here are a few tips to keep them at bay and speed up the healing process:
- Stop smoking.
- Take extra care with your dental hygiene.
- Use a chlorhexidine mouthwash, available from your chemist – this prevents secondary infection and may shorten the episode. However, don't use it long term as it can stain your teeth.
- For pain relief, try applying a salicylic-based gel (available from your chemist) directly on to the ulcer.
- Sucking steroid lozenges at the site of the ulcer also helps relieve pain.
- Applying carmellose paste, again available from your chemist, on to the ulcer, sticks to it and protects it.
- Eat liquorice – it has natural ulcer-healing powers.

GINGIVITIS

This simply means inflamed gums and the most common symptom is gums that bleed when you brush your teeth. It is more common in pregnant women and in people who have diabetes. If the inflammation persists, see your dentist.

MEDICINES AND GINGIVITIS

Some medications cause gingivitis. If your gums start bleeding at the same time as you start a new treatment, it may be worth asking your doctor if you could try an alternative medication. However, you should never stop taking a prescription drug without first discussing it with the doctor who prescribed it.

▼ Brushing your teeth at least twice a day is important in maintaining healthy teeth and gums.

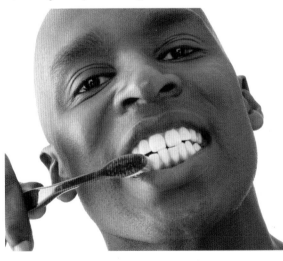

DR DAWN'S HEALTH CHECK
Dental health

You can minimize the risk of gingivitis if you:
- Brush your teeth at least twice a day.
- Floss your teeth each time you brush.
- Have regular dental check-ups and see the hygienist at least twice a year.
- Stop smoking.
- Eat a well-balanced diet.

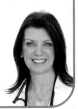

BAD BREATH

Halitosis, or bad breath, affects everyone at some point, but it's a real problem for as many as one in four people. At the risk of stating the obvious, it's important to get a full dental check if you have bad breath – gum disease and tooth decay are some of the main culprits, along with cigarette smoking and excess alcohol intake.

WHAT ELSE CAUSES BAD BREATH?

You would be amazed at the diversity of factors that can cause bad breath. Dieting is a common cause. Other possible explanations include liver or kidney disease. Also some prescribed medications, such as antidepressants, reduce the amount of saliva you produce, which can cause bad breath.

WHAT YOU CAN DO

If this affects you, try chewing sugar-free gum to stimulate saliva production or use an artificial saliva spray, available from your chemist. Good oral hygiene is a must and this doesn't just mean toothbrushing: floss regularly, and visit your dental hygienist every six months to have your gum pockets descaled. It's also worth using a tongue scraper to remove the fur from your tongue. When you first use it you will be appalled by the colour (and smell) of what you remove! If you find you gag when you use it, try doing it at night when your gag reflex is less sensitive. Some people find chewing parsley after meals helps too. Talk to your doctor too, as it's important that medical causes of bad breath are ruled out, or treated.

?
DID YOU KNOW
Mouthwashes

There are many different mouthwashes and all can reduce bad breath temporarily, often by masking the bad breath odour. However, some experts think that mouthwashes may disrupt the normal mouth flora and should not be used as a substitute for proper oral hygiene.

SORE THROAT

The most common reason for someone to make an appointment with his or her doctor is a sore throat; it is also the most likely reason for antibiotics to be prescribed. Tonsillitis is inflammation of the tonsils on either side of the throat, and is one of the commonest causes of a sore throat in children. This occurs because children tend to have prominent tonsils, which are more prone to infection.

HOW SHOULD IT BE TREATED?

The truth is that many sore throats are caused by a viral infection, which can't be treated with antibiotics. Antibiotics are only effective against bacterial infections. Most of us know this on a subconscious level and accept, for example, that a common cold (which is viral) does not need antibiotics; but a sore throat can be confusing. Most sore throats can be treated simply with plenty of fluids, regular paracetamol, and soluble aspirin gargles. These measures will not treat the underlying infection itself but will help to relieve the soreness until the infection clears up.

WHEN DO I NEED ANTIBIOTICS?

How do you know if you have a bacterial infection that needs specific treatment? I tend to make the decision on the duration and severity of symptoms. If your sore throat is getting worse after several days, you have a fever, and you can see yellow pus in the back of your throat, you may well need antibiotics.

My local ear, nose, and throat (ENT) specialist also recommends that anyone who suffers from recurrent sore throats uses a betadine mouthwash, available from your chemist.

WHO NEEDS A TONSILLECTOMY?

When I was a child, it seemed you only had to so much as mention a sore throat and your tonsils were promptly whipped out. Today, far fewer tonsillectomies are performed and this often frustrates parents, who think that doctors are leaving their children to suffer recurrent bouts of tonsillitis.

However, there are reasons for this – studies have shown that removing a child's tonsils achieves an average of only three fewer sore throats in the following two years. Thereafter, children experience the same number of throat infections regardless of whether or not they have their tonsils. Added to that, the fact that most children grow out of the tendency to tonsillitis after the age of about eight, when their throat elongates and the tonsils become less prominent, and a wait-and-see approach starts to make sense.

That said, there is still a place for tonsillectomy. Most doctors will refer a child to an ear, nose, and throat (ENT) specialist if the child has symptoms for more than three months or has had more than five attacks in two years, particularly if they have resulted in the child having to take a lot of time off school. If your child fits into either group, it is worth asking your doctor whether he or she should be referred to a specialist.

▾ *Most sore throats are viral, and can't be treated with antibiotics. It is only if the infection is bacterial that antibiotics should be prescribed.*

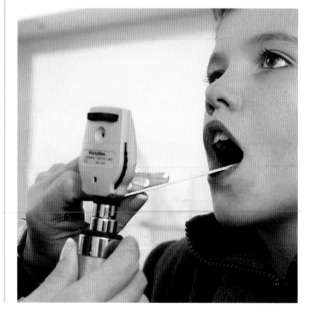

NEURALGIA

One of the major cranial nerves (that supplies sensation to the face, scalp, and mouth), the trigeminal nerve, is sometimes triggered for no apparent reason. This causes a severe burning pain in these areas, which is known as trigeminal neuralgia.

WHAT CAUSES IT?

Doctors don't really know what causes trigeminal neuralgia. Sufferers often find that any stimulation, such as stroking the cheek or even cold wind on the face, can trigger severe pain – so much so that they daren't go outside on cold days.

WHAT YOUR DOCTOR MAY ADVISE

Conventional painkillers are often not enough to control the symptoms and doctors tend to prescribe drugs that stabilize nerve endings, such as antiepileptics and antidepressants, to alleviate the pain. People tend to be frightened of using these drugs, but symptoms can often be controlled on low doses, so they are worth a try.

Some patients also find using a TENS machine, which vibrates on the skin, can help. The theory is that the brain can only cope with a limited number of stimuli at any one time and the vibrations from the TENS machine distract it from concentrating on the facial pain. (TENS machines are so effective that many women use them to alleviate pain during labour).

? DID YOU KNOW
Post-herpetic neuralgia
About 25 per cent of people over 60 who get shingles will develop post-herpetic neuralgia, which can cause burning pain at the site of the shingles rash that lasts long after the rash itself has disappeared. As with trigeminal neuralgia, your doctor may prescribe antidepressant or antiepileptic drugs to relieve the pain of post-herpetic neuralgia.

? DID YOU KNOW
What's in a smile?
Most of us associate smiling with being happy, but have you ever wondered why we sometimes smile when we are unhappy? Back in the 19th century, a French neurologist discovered the difference between the spontaneous and the forced smile. We have all given and received both types of smile – sometimes we are aware of it and sometimes we aren't. So how can you tell the two types of smile apart?

When we smile, the muscles connecting the cheeks and the corners of the lips contract, pulling the mouth into a smile. We have voluntary control over these muscles so can force a smile even if we don't feel particularly happy; this is called a non-D smile. A broad non-D smile might also produce wrinkling around the eyes but no dipping of the eyebrows. When we are genuinely happy, the muscles around the eyes also contract, causing laughter lines and a slight dipping of the eyebrows; this is the D smile. So the clue is all in the eyebrows, and it's almost impossible to cheat – most of us have no voluntary control over these muscles!

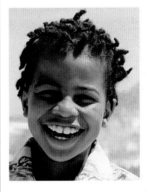

◄ *A real smile, showing wrinkling around the eyes and a slight dipping of the eyebrows.*

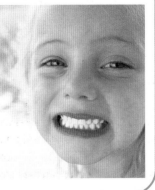

A fake smile, with wrinkling around the eyes but no dipping of the eyebrows. ▶

• There are around 100,000 to 150,000 hairs on an average scalp • You lose up to 100 hairs a day without really noticing; this is the normal hair loss you see in your hairbrush or in the plughole • Hair grows about 1cm (½in) a month • Each hair grows for around five years before it falls out, and each hair follicle produces about 20 hairs in its lifetime • At any one time, ten per cent of your hair will be in a resting phase – this lasts for between two and three months before the hair goes through a shedding phase • Straight hair is round in cross-section, wavy hair is alternately round and oval.

2

Hair

Introduction Maintaining a healthy head of hair is a huge industry. Whether we perm, colour, or simply have it regularly cut, most of us will spend several thousand pounds in our lifetime on looking after our hair. And as we get older, we find ourselves spending more and more as we strive to hide the nasty way our hair has of giving away our age!

Apart from the soles of our feet and the palms of our hands, hair grows all over our bodies. Much of it is finer and less obvious in women than it is in men, as the higher levels of testosterone in men trigger a change in body hair follicles, causing them to grow thicker, longer, and often darker body hair. In men and women body hair grows more slowly than scalp hair, and each hair grows for only around three months before it enters its static phase and is then shed.

The length of time that our hair continues to produce pigment is genetically programmed, and at some point in the ageing process we all gradually lose the colour.

HAIR LOSS

Concerns over hair loss are a common complaint in my surgery. Often it's simply a part of the natural ageing process, but there are several things that can cause us to lose our hair which we can do something about.

HAIR LOSS AND HORMONES

A common cause of hair loss is increased sensitivity to hormones, and it's not just men who suffer. Hormones cause hair thinning in one in ten women under 40 and a quarter of all women over 50. But, interestingly, the way we lose our hair in response to hormones tends to differ between the sexes: men develop a bald crown and/or a receding hairline; women usually lose hair more diffusely, giving a generalized thinning rather than a bald patch. The menopause can also cause hair loss – sometimes this can be helped by hormone replacement therapy (HRT).

Daily applications of minoxidil lotion, available from your chemist, can help stimulate hair growth, but it only works while it is being used and it can cause unwanted facial hair in women.

DOES DIET MAKE A DIFFERENCE?

In animals, hair is needed to maintain body temperature, but in humans it is not essential. As a result, if you don't eat enough, your body will tend to lose hair quickly. Any low-calorie, low-protein diet can cause hair loss, which is why most anorexics have thinning hair.

The mineral iron (found most commonly in green leafy vegetables and red meat) is particularly important for the maintenance of healthy hair. We can measure iron levels (ferritin) in the blood – a level over 10 is considered normal, and below that you may be at risk of anaemia (see p.61). However, I aim for a level of over 70 in anyone who has problems with hair loss. Although I am generally not keen on iron supplements, in these cases they may be necessary to achieve such an increase.

EFFECTS OF STRESS

I have no doubt that stress can cause hair loss – we have all heard stories of people who experience a tragedy and lose their hair overnight. It happens, but thankfully very rarely. Much more common is the more diffuse thinning as a result of stress – and there is science behind it: high stress levels are associated with high levels of the hormone prolactin, which affects the way we metabolize testosterone (women produce small amounts of testosterone too). Stress may also contribute to hair loss by reducing blood flow to the scalp.

WHAT ELSE CAUSES HAIR LOSS?

As well as stress and ageing, hair loss can be caused by traction (tight ponytails or over-use of hair straighteners), hair dyes, and chemical treatments such as bleaching.

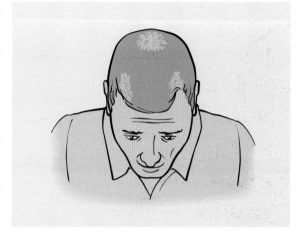

▲ Hair loss in men tends to occur as a bald patch on the crown and/or a receding hairline.

▼ Hair loss in women generally occurs as a generalized thinning over the whole scalp.

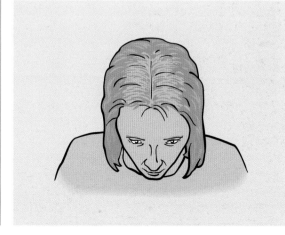

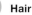
Any severe illness can be associated with hair loss, and everyone knows that chemotherapy treatment for cancer often causes dramatic loss of hair, but there are other conditions and drugs that could also be to blame, including:

• Skin diseases such as eczema or psoriasis.
• Diabetes (see p.101).
• Hypothyroidism (underactivity of the thyroid gland).
• Burns or severe injury.
• Some blood-thinning drugs (anticoagulants) and antidepressants – although you should never stop taking any prescribed medication without checking with your doctor. If all other possible causes of hair loss have been ruled out, it's worth asking whether there are any suitable alternative medications.

? **DID YOU KNOW**

Why do new mothers lose masses of hair?

Hormonal changes when you are pregnant stop the hair from entering its shedding phase so you no longer lose the 100 hairs or so each day that constitutes normal hair loss – this is also one reason why pregnant women often 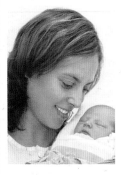 seem to have thicker, healthier-looking hair. After your baby is born, hormone levels drop dramatically and all the hairs that would have fallen out while you were pregnant fall out at the same time; typically from about three to six months after the birth. (Occasionally this happens to women who stop taking the combined contraceptive pill.) Losing a year's worth of hair in a short period of time is distressing, and I probably see at least one new mother every month who is convinced she is going to be bald by the end of the year. Your hair will return to normal, although it can take several months for this to happen.

ALOPECIA AREATA

Alopecia is an umbrella term that is used to describe patchy hair loss. It occurs in about one per cent of the population and may involve the whole scalp (when it is known as alopecia totalis) or, more rarely, all body and facial hair (alopecia universalis).

WHAT CAUSES IT?

Alopecia is a genetic condition (20 per cent of patients have a relative with the problem), but genes aren't the whole story and often the hair loss is triggered by an infection or emotional stress. The younger you are when you develop the condition, the greater the risk of its progressing to alopecia totalis or universalis – half of those who develop alopecia before puberty will go on to develop the most severe form (alopecia universalis).

WILL MY HAIR GROW BACK?

It can be difficult to predict the course of alopecia. Many people return to normal, but it can take months or years. However, you are less likely to regain a full head of hair if:

• You develop alopecia before puberty.
• Hair loss persists for more than a year.
• You have had previous attacks.
• You lose your eyebrows and eyelashes.
• You have another associated illness, such as thyroid disease or eczema.

▼ *A bald patch on the scalp characteristic of alopecia.*

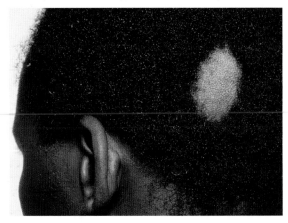

TRICHOTILLOMANIA

Quite literally, trichotillomania means the compulsion to pull out your hair, and while most people may never have heard the term, the condition is surprisingly common – according to the support group, one in ten people may suffer from it to some degree.

WHAT CAUSES IT?
The first episodes of trichotillomania are often triggered by acute stress – the loss of a parent or a disturbed parent-child relationship are classic examples. Most sufferers try to hide their actions, then develop problems with feelings of guilt and low self-esteem.

WHAT ARE THE SYMPTOMS?
Most sufferers pull out hair from the scalp, but around one in four pull out their eyebrows or eyelashes and one in five will pull out both, while a minority, less than one in ten, pull out hair from other parts of their body. The average age of onset is 12 years, but it can happen later. You may notice a member of your family tugging at their hair, particularly during times of stress. More commonly, you may see bald patches starting to appear, especially around the temples.

WHAT YOU CAN DO
Recognizing that there is a problem is the first step to getting better. It is helpful if the sufferer has somebody to confide in – there's a lot of truth in the old saying "a problem shared is a problem halved". Dealing with any underlying stress is an important part of treatment and many patients benefit from one of the talking therapies, such as cognitive behavioural therapy. Your family doctor can recommend local services.

FIND OUT MORE
www.trichotillomania.co.uk

DANDRUFF

This occurs when the scalp begins to flake and small white scales form in your hair. It is more common in men than women, and is usually caused by a yeast infection. Yeasts thrive in warm, moist environments, which explains why dandruff seems to reach a peak at the age of 20, when we produce a natural oil in our scalp called sebum.

WHAT YOU CAN DO
Wash your hair once or twice a week with a medicated shampoo that contains selenium sulphide, pyrithione zinc, or tar extracts – ask your pharmacist for advice. In resistant cases, I recommend trying an antifungal shampoo. These can be bought over the counter, but if they don't seem to work, have a chat with your doctor as he or she may be able to prescribe something stronger. When the dandruff is under control, you may be able to return to your original shampoo, but be prepared to use a medicated shampoo every couple of weeks to prevent the dandruff recurring.

▼ *Using a medicated shampoo once or twice a week can help to keep dandruff under control.*

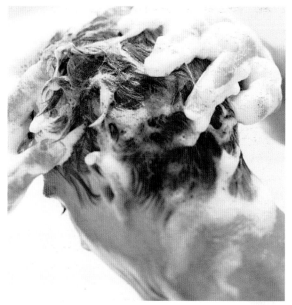

EXCESS HAIR

At least 25 per cent of middle-aged women have some unwanted facial hair and this increases as they get older. For most, it is just a family trait – if your mother had a lot of excess hair then the odds are you will too, but there can be other causes.

WHAT CAUSES IT

- Ethnicity – excess hair (hirsutism) is common in dark-haired women, particularly those of Mediterranean or Asian origin.
- Polycystic ovary syndrome (PCOS; see p.145) – this is a hormonal condition characterized by excess hair growth, weight gain, and irregular periods. Losing weight can help reduce the excess hair, but can be difficult.
- Medication – some antiepileptic drugs and steroids may cause excess hair growth and it can take a year or more to return to normal after stopping the drug.
- Tumours – thankfully these are rare, but tumours of the ovary or adrenal gland can cause excessive body hair.

WHAT YOU CAN DO

Excess hair can cause immense distress, particularly to women. A whole industry has arisen out of the need to remove or hide unwanted hair. The options include:

- Bleaching – you can apply special bleach, available from the chemist, to hide the excess hair.
- Shaving – contrary to popular belief, shaving doesn't encourage hairs to grow back more quickly; electric shavers probably damage the skin less than wet shaving.
- Depilatory creams – although some creams cause a skin reaction, and the hair grows back.
- Plucking – can be painful, and the hair regrows.
- Waxing – like the other methods here, the hair regrows.
- Electrolysis – unlike all the options above, this can permanently remove hair but can only be done on small areas at a time so is time-consuming and expensive. In unskilled hands it can cause scarring – always check your therapist's qualifications.
- Laser – like electrolysis, laser treatment can remove hair permanently but it is expensive. It is less painful than electrolysis and works best on dark hair. Always check your therapist's qualifications.

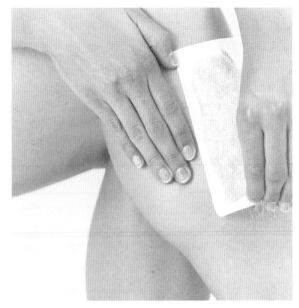

▲ *Waxing removes hair for several weeks at a time, but it doesn't suit everyone.*

DR DAWN'S HEALTH CHECK
Pros and cons of the treatments

Which method of hair removal you choose will depend on personal preference and budget, but the following tips may help you to decide:

- Bleaching is good if you have a small amount of unwanted dark hair but is not really satisfactory if you have a lot of unwanted hair, and it can also cause irritation of the skin.
- Shaving and depilatory creams are cheap but hair removal needs to be repeated quite frequently.
- Waxing gives a slightly longer-term result but some women (particularly those with dark hair, which tends to be coarser) develop problems with hair growing back under the top layer of skin. These ingrowing hairs may make you prone to boils; gently rubbing off the top layer of skin daily with a loofah may help.
- Electrolysis removes unwanted hair permanently but is unsuitable for large areas, and is time-consuming and relatively expensive.
- Laser treatment can remove hair permanently (although there may be some hair regrowth), and can be used on any part of the body. It doesn't work on white, grey, or blonde hair, and it is expensive.

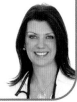

MYTH BUSTERS
Let's take a look at some of the myths that we hear about hair.

BALDNESS IS RELATED TO TESTOSTERONE LEVELS	TRUE	Male baldness is linked to hypersensitivity of hair follicles to the male hormone testosterone. Hair loss in women is also linked to hormone disturbances, especially after the menopause.
BALDNESS IN A MAN IS INHERITED ONLY FROM HIS MOTHER	FALSE	Sorry guys – it's not just your mother. Hereditary factors linked to premature balding are usually passed down from your mother, but hair loss in your father also plays a significant role in increasing the likelihood of going bald.
SHAVING MAKES HAIR GROW BACK MORE THICKLY	FALSE	It won't make the hair grow back thicker, but unfortunately it will grow back.
A BABY DEVELOPS A BALD PATCH ON THE BACK OF HIS OR HER HEAD FROM RUBBING ON THE MATTRESS	FALSE	All babies start to shed their first hair at two to three months; this is replaced by a second growth. The hair loss does start at the back of the head but it has nothing to do with friction.
GREY HAIR IS HEREDITARY	TRUE	As you age, the cells that produce pigment stop working and hair loses its natural colouring. The lifespan of these cells is largely determined by genes, so if your parents went grey in their thirties then you may well follow suit.
SMOKING CAUSES PREMATURE GREYING	TRUE	Smokers do tend to go grey earlier. One theory is that smoking affects the scalp's blood supply so the pigment-producing cells don't work as well.
PLUCKING ONE GREY HAIR RESULTS IN TWO MORE GROWING BACK	FALSE	It just seems like it!
HAIR DYES CAUSE CANCER	TRUE POSSIBLY	This is a controversial area but one study in America showed that women who used permanent hair dyes were three times more likely to develop bladder cancer than those who didn't. It's only one study, but it's enough for me to stick to semi-permanent dyes.
BALDNESS IS LINKED TO IQ	FALSE	This is an urban myth that I suspect has its roots in an attempt to put a positive spin on going bald, but there is no truth in the idea that intelligent men are more likely to go bald.

• Your skin has phenomenal powers of regeneration, and completely replaces itself every two months • Every 1cm^2 (½in^2) of skin contains 3,000,000 cells, 10 hairs, 200 pain receptors, 25 pressure sensors, 3,000 nerve endings, and 100 sweat glands • Sweat glands in our skin can produce an incredible two litres of sweat in just one hour when exercising hard in a hot environment • Around 1,600 nerves detect heat and cold, but around four million are responsible for the sensation of touch, and the impulses from these nerves travel back to the brain at over 250 km/h.

3

Skin

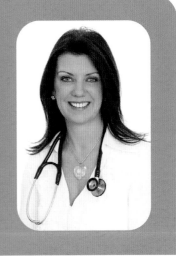

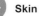

Introduction Your skin is the largest organ in your body, and there is a lot more to it than you might realize – without it you would die. The surface area of skin for the average adult is around 2m^2 (22ft^2); skin accounts for almost one sixth of your body weight. Its thickness varies from just ½mm on your eyelids to about 4mm (⅙in) or more on the palms of your hands or soles of your feet.

Skin has two layers – the outer epidermis, and the inner dermis. It's main function is to protect your body from pollutants, ultraviolet rays, and infections. It is basically a waterproof wrapping that prevents you from drying up! Skin is in direct contact with the outside world, and by a series of complex messages that pass between its receptors and the brain, it is responsible for fine-tuning your body temperature.

Your skin is an amazing organ, but there is a lot that can go wrong with it – around one in ten doctor's appointments are for skin-related conditions.

ECZEMA

This is a common skin condition that affects as many as one in five children and between two and ten per cent of the adult population. The good news is that around one third of children with eczema will grow out of it by their mid-teens.

FEATURES OF ECZEMA

The main features of eczema are dryness and inflammation, resulting in very itchy skin. I am often asked about the difference between eczema and dermatitis, but to be honest, the two terms are interchangeable. The most common forms of ezcema are listed below.

COMMON FORMS OF ECZEMA

• Atopic eczema is the most common form of eczema. It often tends to run in families, and is closely linked to asthma and hayfever.

• Allergic contact dermatitis results from an allergic reaction to a substance in contact with the skin, such as contact with rings, watch straps, and belt buckles.

• Irritant contact dermatitis is an irritation caused by frequent contact with chemicals; I often see this type of dermatitis on the hands of hairdressers.

• Infantile seborrhoeic eczema is also known as cradle cap, and is a condition that occurs in babies. It can look unpleasant but it's rarely itchy and usually clears up within a few months.

▼ *Atopic eczema typically develops in skin creases, such as the backs of the knees and insides of the elbows.*

CAN IT BE CURED?

There is currently no cure for eczema, but researchers have identified a gene responsible for producing a protective protein that is defective in eczema sufferers. This discovery could herald the development of a whole new way of treating the condition, but in the meantime we have to treat the symptoms as they arise and avoid any triggers that may cause the condition to flare up.

DR DAWN'S HEALTH CHECK
Dos and don'ts for eczema

As with so many skin conditions, there is a lot of confusion about what is good and bad for eczema sufferers, so here's a list of my recommendations.

Do:

• Use emollients – these help prevent drying of the skin. They can be used directly on the skin at least twice a day, as a soap substitute, and in the bath.

• Use steroids as prescribed by your doctor – they are perfectly safe as long as they are used appropriately. As a rough guide, you should be applying ten times as much emollient as steroid.

• Avoid extremes of temperature – hot and cold temperatures can both irritate the skin.

• Keep nails short – scratching is often worse at night. Cotton gloves or mittens, available from your chemist, may help reduce damage to the skin from scratching.

• Keep a food diary – diet is often blamed for eczema, although food is the main trigger in only one in ten children. Exclude those foods that clearly exacerbate it, but take the advice of a dietitian.

• Consult your doctor if the condition flares up.

Don't:

• Use soap – it dries the skin and makes eczema worse.

• Use perfumed bubble baths – these also dry the skin.

• Use aerosol deodorants – alcohol-free roll-on deodorants are less likely to cause irritation.

• Rub the skin dry after bathing – patting the skin dry is less irritant.

• Overuse steroid creams – the amount of cream you can put on the tip of your finger is enough to cover an area twice the size of the palm of your hand.

WHAT YOUR DOCTOR MAY ADVISE

Your doctor may advise a combination of emollients – creams that moisturize the skin and prevent it from becoming too dry – and steroid creams to reduce inflammation. In some cases, your doctor may prescribe antibiotics if the skin becomes infected.

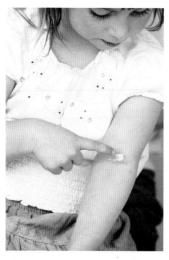

Emolllient creams applied to the affected areas of skin can help prevent dryness. ▸

FIND OUT MORE
www.eczema.org

PSORIASIS

This is a chronic (long-term) condition in which the skin cells regenerate 20 times faster than normal, producing red patches of skin with a characteristic silver scaling; these patches are called plaques. The plaques occur most commonly on the knees, elbows, and scalp.

WHAT CAUSES IT?

Psoriasis affects about two per cent of the population. It usually starts before the age of 40, and in one third of cases another member of the family is also affected. We don't fully understand why psoriasis develops, but stress (physical or emotional) and infections can play an important part in the condition. About ten per cent of people with psoriasis also develop arthritis, typically in the fingers or spine.

WHAT YOUR DOCTOR MAY ADVISE

There is no cure for psoriasis, but there are lots of options available to keep it under control. Emollients and bath additives moisturize the skin and reduce the discomfort of the scaling. In most cases, psoriasis is managed with the treatments described below but more severe cases will be referred to a specialist, who may prescribe oral medication or ultraviolet light therapy.

PSORIASIS TREATMENTS

• Coal tar – this comes in different concentrations, from one to ten per cent, and is applied topically. However, coal tar preparations are messy and stain clothing so are only used at home for small patches of psoriasis; patients with larger areas that need treatment are usually admitted to hospital.

• Dithranol paste – this is an effective topical treatment but it may cause staining of the skin. It needs to be left on for 30 minutes and then be washed off to avoid irritating the normal underlying skin.

• Steroids – strong steroid creams are often needed and there is a marked improvement within four weeks in around half of patients.

• Vitamin D analogues – lotions that are simple to use, but some people become resistant to them over time.

▾ *Psoriasis causes red, scaly patches due to the skin regenerating much faster than normal.*

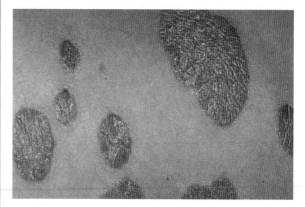

FIND OUT MORE
www.psoriasis-association.org.uk

ACNE

Around eight out of ten teenagers suffer from acne, a condition in which spots develop on the skin. The spots are caused by overstimulation of the sebaceous glands in the skin, which produce an oily substance called sebum. The sebum blocks the pores and makes people prone to spots.

TEENAGE ACNE

Teenage acne is associated with a rise in the levels of the male hormone testosterone as puberty is reached. Whether or not you develop spots has nothing to do with how high the testosterone levels are, it depends on the sensitivity of your skin to the hormone – and girls produce testosterone too. It is the testosterone that stimulates the glands to produce sebum, blocking pores and causing spots.

ADULT ACNE

The good news is that most people grow out of it by their late teens or early twenties. However, a few people will still be struggling with it into their forties. There is also an adult form called acne rosacea that affects one in ten women between the ages of 30 and 50. It can affect men too, although it's less common. In both men and women it tends to run in families. Acne rosacea causes red skin with broken veins and acne-like pustules on the forehead, cheeks, and nose.

WHAT YOU CAN DO

Chemists' shelves are packed with products claiming to clear your skin. I find the most effective are creams that contain benzoyl peroxide. These creams come in varying strengths so always try the weakest first; ask your pharmacist for advice.

Soap can alter the pH of the skin and in some people may make acne worse. Try washing your skin with an antiseptic solution (ten parts water to one part antiseptic) instead; it can really help control greasy skin.

WHAT YOUR DOCTOR MAY ADVISE

If over-the-counter remedies don't work, don't despair. Your doctor will be able to help. It's such a common problem that I see someone with acne almost every day. My first line is to try topical antibiotics, such as creams or gels, some of which contain vitamin A. If they don't work, it may be worth trying a course of antibiotics. These are normally taken every day for several months. It often takes eight weeks or so to see a definite improvement.

One type of oral contraceptive (Co-cyprindiol) is also licensed for the treatment of acne. It is very effective, although it is not suitable for all women. In very severe cases, I refer patients to a consultant dermatologist, because there are some treatments that are only available via a specialist.

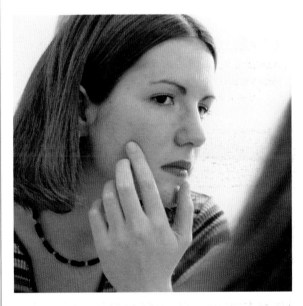

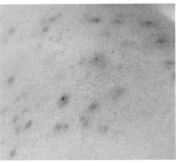

▲ ◄ Acne causes blocked pores and spots, and eight out of ten teenagers will suffer from it at some point.

FIND OUT MORE
www.stopspots.org

MYTH BUSTERS
There are numerous myths about acne so let's take a look at some of them.

EATING CHOCOLATE MAKES ACNE WORSE — FALSE

Years of research have failed to show any link between acne and diet. A balanced diet promotes healthy skin but if your children want chocolate from time to time, it won't give them spots.

SQUEEZING BLACKHEADS WILL GET RID OF THEM MORE QUICKLY — FALSE

Squeezing spots and blackheads can force the contents deeper into the skin and cause scarring. The best way to remove blackheads is with a comedone spoon available from chemists. Alternatively, you can use the side of your thumb and the soft tip of a finger. Never use your nails – you could scar your face.

GREASY MOISTURIZERS MAKE ACNE WORSE — TRUE

Greasy moisturizers and make-up can block pores and cause spots. Acne sufferers should stick to oil-free products.

ACNE CREAMS CLEAR UP SPOTS — FALSE

Most acne treatments are aimed at preventing new spots not curing existing ones, so it's important to use them on any areas that may be susceptible.

HAIR PRODUCTS CAUSE ACNE — TRUE

Some defrizzing products can cause an outcrop of acne along the hairline.

ACNE RUNS IN FAMILIES — TRUE

Acne isn't strictly genetic but if you suffered, then your children are more likely to, although there is no link between how severe your acne may have been and what will happen to them.

ACNE IS A SIGN OF POOR PERSONAL HYGIENE — FALSE

The black of blackheads is due to the pigment of the cells blocking the pores – it isn't dirt. In fact, overzealous washing or scrubbing can make acne worse. Ideally, you should wash your face with an antiseptic solution (see p.37) using your hands, not a flannel, and pat your skin dry.

PERIODS MAKE ACNE WORSE — TRUE

Acne sufferers often find their spots are worse just before a period. This is thought to be due to hormonal changes.

GREASY HAIR CAUSES ACNE — FALSE

Greasy hair doesn't cause acne but people with greasy hair often have oily skin and are therefore more prone to acne. Your acne will respond to normal measures regardless of your hair.

SUNLIGHT HELPS ACNE — TRUE

The ultraviolet rays in sunlight can help dry up spots but there is a fine line here. Sweating can clog up pores, which can lead to a new set of spots developing.

BOILS

A boil is an abscess in the skin that usually develops in a hair follicle or sweat gland. Pus collects, causing a red, painful lump; if left, the lump may develop a head and then rupture, discharging the pus.

WHAT CAUSES THEM?

Boils are most commonly found on the face and hairline, especially on areas that you shave. Anywhere that hairs may grow back into the skin is more prone to boils. Some people find that removing hair by waxing also makes them more prone to boils, as the hairs often regrow under the skin. Exfoliating your skin daily using a loofah or skin scrub may help to prevent boils forming, but you may need to consider another form of hair removal if the problem persists.

WHEN YOU SHOULD SEE A DOCTOR

After a boil has discharged its pus, the pain is often less because the pressure has been relieved. However, you should still see your doctor as you probably need antibiotics to clear the infection and reduce the risk of recurrence. If you suffer frequent attacks of boils, you should see your doctor to rule out diabetes (see p.101).

▾ *Although boils are not serious, if they develop on a bony area the surrounding skin can become very tense and painful.*

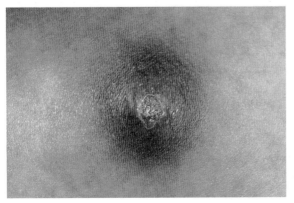

WARTS

Many people (especially children) get warts at some time. They are caused by the human papillomavirus, of which there are around 100 types (see also Verrucas, p.134). All warts will disappear eventually but they usually persist for several months, and occasionally for two or three years.

SHOULD THEY BE TREATED?

Generally, people put up with warts, at least for the first few weeks, but I am often asked about them because people are fed up with waiting for them to go. Advocates of "leave nature to its course" argue that by allowing the wart to run its natural course the body mounts an immune response to them; this could explain why warts are more common in children. Also, warts rarely cause any problems other than being unsightly. In most cases, I agree with the wait-and-see approach – many of the treatments are at best uncomfortable and at worse painful. However, if a wart is troubling you by being too unsightly, try the measures described below.

WHAT YOU CAN DO

You can try filing down the wart with a pumice stone, applying a salicylate-based paint (available from your chemist), then covering it with duct tape. You will need to be patient though – the process needs repeating daily and it can take several weeks for the wart to disappear.

Some people recommend using tea-tree oil – again, pare down the wart slightly, then apply a small amount of concentrated oil every night until the wart has gone. This method isn't scientifically proven, but it's less painful than the medical alternative, cryotherapy, which involves freezing the wart and underlying tissues.

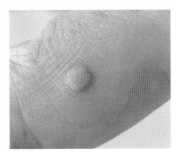

◄ *Warts can be unsightly but are rarely serious.*

EXCESSIVE SWEATING

Known as hyperhidrosis, excessive sweating affects at least one in 100 people in the UK, with most sufferers being in their twenties or thirties. The armpits, hands, and feet are the areas most commonly affected.

WHAT YOU CAN DO

The problem is typically made worse by stress and you can enter a vicious cycle – the more you sweat, the more you worry, and vice versa. Step one is to use a medical-grade roll-on antiperspirant (available without prescription from your chemist). They are a lot more powerful than conventional antiperspirants. You apply them before going to bed at night, and wash them off in the morning.

WHAT YOUR DOCTOR MAY ADVISE

If a medical-grade antiperspirant doesn't work, ask your doctor about injections of botulinum toxin into the armpits, which sounds awful but is very effective. The treatment involves lots of tiny injections into the skin of your armpits – it's so effective, it's like turning off a tap. However, the effect lasts only for about six months. As a last resort, you can have the nerves to the sweat glands cut (an operation called a sympathectomy).

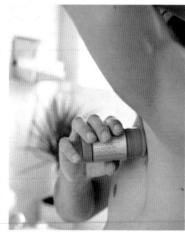

Medical-grade antiperspirants can reduce excessive sweating. ▸

FIND OUT MORE
www.sweating.co.uk

BODY ODOUR

Fresh sweat doesn't have a particular odour, but when it is broken down by bacteria that live naturally on the skin, it can develop that characteristic strong smell that people can find offensive.

WHAT YOU CAN DO

There are a few simple things you can do at home. The skin in the armpit has a natural pH of about 6.5 and this mildly acidic environment prevents the growth of bacteria on the skin. Normal soap is alkaline (about pH10) and it can take up to 12 hours for your skin to regain its natural acidity after you use soap, allowing the bacteria to multiply. Using a pH-balanced soap helps keep the bacteria in check.

The average body has two million sweat glands, and the glands in the armpits alone can produce more than 11 litres (about 20 pints) of sweat in 24 hours. Hairy armpits can retain 30 times more sweat than hairless ones, so shaving or waxing will help reduce odour.

Wash your clothes regularly, and never wear yesterday's socks or underwear. Strongly perfumed products are likely to adversely alter the skin pH too, so stick to using unperfumed, pH-balanced products.

 DR DAWN'S HEALTH CHECK
If someone else has body odour

One of the problems with body odour is that, because it develops insidiously, a person may not be aware that he or she has it – I have often heard it described as the condition even your best friend won't tell you that you have. But a good friend must say something.

• Don't avoid the subject – it's not an easy subject to broach, but just think how much you would hate it to be you that suffered while others talked behind your back.

• Be sensitive and pick your moment – this is not a talk to have in public.

• Offer practical advice on how to deal with it – now that you have read this you will have some useful tips!

SUN AND THE SKIN

The sun's rays contain two types of ultraviolet light – UVA and UVB. Both damage the skin, and the fairer our skin, the more susceptible we are to the harmful effects of exposure to sunlight.

THE EFFECTS OF SUN EXPOSURE ON SKIN

The top layer of skin absorbs 90 per cent of the UVB rays (which can lead to sunburn), and therefore only ten per cent of UVB rays reach the underlying dermis. On the other hand, all of the UVA rays reach the dermis, where they damage the connective tissues, causing wrinkles and premature ageing. Both UVA and UVB have been implicated as causes of skin cancer. Sunbeds use predominantly UVA, so although you may not get burned, you may still damage your skin.

THE RIGHT SUNSCREEN IS IMPORTANT

Choose your sunscreen carefully. The sun-protection factor (SPF) tends to refer to protection from UVB while a star-rating tells you how much protection you will get from UVA. Ideally, you should opt for a high SPF with a 3 or 4 star-rating. The sunscreen should be at least SPF 15, and SPF 30 for fair-skinned people. It should be applied generously and frequently.

▼ *It's really important to protect children from the damaging effects of the sun. Always use a high-factor sun screen (factor 15+), and use hats and protective clothing when necessary.*

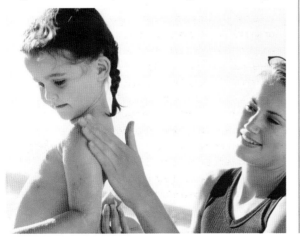

Sometimes, it can be difficult to judge the strength of the sun. Looking up the UV index helps; it is shown in a triangle on the weather forecast. Between October and March in the UK the index is rarely over 3 and even the fairest skins are safe, but at the height of summer it can reach 7, when you will need to use sunscreen.

HOW SHOULD I TREAT SUNBURN?

It is better to prevent sunburn in the first place but if you have been burned, make sure you drink plenty of cool fluids, take a tepid bath or shower, and remove any excess clothing. Calamine lotion may also help soothe the skin, or apply a moisturizer to help rehydrate the skin.

DR DAWN'S HEALTH CHECK
Protecting children's skin

Children and people with fair skin are most at risk and need the most protection. It has been estimated that most of us have had 80 per cent of our lifetime exposure to sun by the age of 21, and children's skin is more vulnerable to its damaging effects because it is thinner and the layers of pigment are not as well developed.

• Wherever possible, children under a year should stay in the shade, especially during the hottest part of the day.
• Using a wide-brimmed hat on your child will protect his or her face and the back of the neck.
• Use the sunshade on your buggy.
• Get your child to wear UV-resistant clothing, if possible.
• Remember when buying sunglasses that you get what you pay for. I know children lose sunglasses, but it is still worth buying good-quality glasses with guaranteed UV protection. Without the UV protection, a child's eyes are not protected even if the lenses are dark. In fact, they can allow the pupil to dilate in bright light, thus exposing the retina to more rays.
• Always apply factor 15+ sunscreen before children go outdoors, and reapply often to be sure of good coverage.

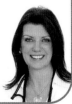

FIND OUT MORE
www.sunsmart.org.uk

SKIN CANCER

This is one of the most common forms of cancer in the UK and the number of cases is increasing every year. The single biggest risk factor is exposure to sunlight. Just one episode of sunburn as a child doubles your risk of skin cancer later in life.

TYPES OF SKIN CANCER

There are three main types of skin cancer: basal cell cancers, squamous cell cancers, and melanomas. The first two often occur on areas of the skin that have had a lot of sun exposure – typically the face and hands. They tend to be slow-growing and can usually be treated relatively easily. It is often possible to remove such tumours surgically – especially if they are treated in the early stages – although radiotherapy (or, rarely, chemotherapy) may sometimes be necessary.

DR DAWN'S HEALTH CHECK
Preventing skin cancer

You can reduce your and your family's risk of developing skin cancer if you:

• Use a high SPF sunscreen and apply it thickly enough – a 200ml (7fl oz) bottle should provide you with around six full-body applications. Reapply it every two hours, and always after swimming.

• Remember that sunscreen has a shelf life, so don't use anything that has been in the back of the cupboard for 10 years! It needs to be replaced at least every 2–3 years. Never use a sunscreen after its use-by date, and store it in a cool place out of direct sunlight.

• Don't use a lower SPF sunscreen if you have a tan – a tan simply means that your skin has been damaged by the sun and is producing pigment to try to protect itself. Experts believe that the protective power of a tan is only as strong as SPF 2–4 sunscreen.

• Stay out of the sun between 11am and 3pm, when the sun is at its strongest. If in doubt, look at your shadow – if it's shorter than you, the sun is strong enough for you to need to protect your skin.

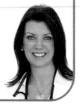

• Avoid using sunbeds.

Melanomas are the most dangerous type because they can spread rapidly to other parts of the body, which may be fatal. They can occur anywhere on the body and develop after high-intensity sun exposure rather than long-term, low-grade exposure. A melanoma may appear as a new mole or one that is changing. Treatment is usually by surgery, but radiotherapy and/or chemotherapy may also be needed, especially if the cancer has spread.

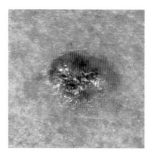

◀ *A basal cell cancer typically first appears as a small, painless lump.*

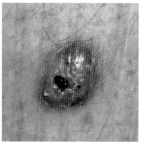

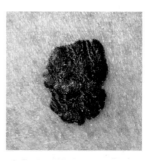

▲ *A squamous cancer usually appears as a red lump that later ulcerates.*

◀ *A melanoma is usually dark with an irregular edge.*

! SEEK MEDICAL ADVICE NOW
If you notice a mole change in any of the following ways:

• It changes shape.
• It changes colour.
• It is getting bigger.
• It begins to itch.
• It begins to bleed.
• New moles develop around it.

FIND OUT MORE
www.skincancer.org

VITILIGO

This condition produces patches of white skin that don't contain normal skin pigment. These patches are often found on the face and hands, and can be more noticeable if you have darker skin.

WHAT CAUSES IT?

Vitiligo occurs when the top layers of the skin stop producing the pigment melanin. The underlying cause is not properly understood, but it is estimated that vitiligo affects one in 100 adults in the UK. Although it can start at any age, 50 per cent of people with vitiligo develop it before the age of 25.

WHAT YOU CAN DO

Patches of vitiligo don't have any protection against the sun, so it is important to use a high-protection sunscreen (SPF 20+). Avoiding exposure to the sun may help to keep the patchy appearance to a minimum. Camouflage make-up can also be effective – many areas now run camouflage clinics that can provide special make-up on prescription, so it may be worth talking to your doctor about this. Paradoxically, light therapy may also be effective, although this is a long-term treatment.

▼ *Patches of depigmentation caused by vitiligo.*

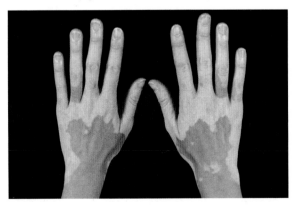

FIND OUT MORE
www.vitiligosociety.org.uk

TATTOOS

These have become very popular in recent years but I must add a word of caution – there is undoubtedly a risk of infection with serious viruses, including HIV and hepatitis, if the salon is not scrupulous about sterilizing equipment. In addition, there is also a risk of bacterial infection, which can leave permanent scarring.

CAN THEY BE REMOVED?

I am often asked about this. The answer is that the fine lines blur over time; laser techniques can help but they can be expensive. Lasers work best on the blue/black inks but don't usually manage to obliterate tattoos completely. So think hard before having a tattoo – it might be there for life. Henna tattoos are a good alternative and will fade over time. Some transfers look just as good as real tattoos and they don't carry any of the risks.

BODY PIERCING

Body piercing has been practised as far back as it is possible to trace. It has usually been confined to the ears, mouth, and nose, but now the most popular sites are the nipples and belly button. I have seen lots of belly buttons infected after piercing, most of which require antibiotics.

WHAT TO DO IF YOU GET AN INFECTION

A mild infection will sometimes clear up if you clean the area daily with an antiseptic solution, such as four per cent chorhexidine gluconate (available from your chemist). You should also avoid tight clothing that rubs against the infected piercing. It is usually best to keep the ring in place because it helps allow the infection to drain. If the infection hasn't cleared up within a few days, you should see your doctor, who will probably prescribe antibiotics. However, if the infection persists after the course of antibiotics, you may need to consider changing to a better-quality piece of jewellery, or even removing the ring entirely for a while.

• Your heart beats around 40 to 50 million times a year and never takes a rest • Every year your heart pumps over three million litres (five million pints) of blood through your body and an equal amount through your lungs • Our hearts pump blood through 100,000km (62,000 miles) of blood vessels • Our heart muscle is unique – it contracts rhythmically all day and night under autonomic, or reflex, control; unlike the muscles in our arms and legs, we have no voluntary control over it • Your heart has its own built-in pacemaker that fires about 72 electrical impulses into the muscles every minute.

4

Heart & circulation

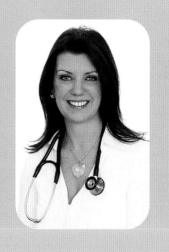

Introduction The heart is the most important muscle in the body – if it stops working we die. The heart is the pump that sends the fuel to all parts of our bodies. It is made up of four chambers – two on the left and two on the right. The left side of the heart receives blood rich in oxygen from our lungs into a chamber called the left atrium. Blood then passes through a one-way valve into the biggest chamber of the heart, the left ventricle, into blood vessels called arteries from where the blood is pumped out to our brain, gut, kidneys, liver, and limbs, as well of course as the heart muscle itself (via coronary arteries).

The right side of the heart receives the blood back from the body into the right atrium from vessels called veins. By the time blood reaches the right atrium, the oxygen has been removed and the blood is carrying waste products, including carbon dioxide, to be expelled from the body. Blood then passes through another one-way valve into the right ventricle before being pumped to the lungs. The carbon dioxide passes into the lungs to be breathed out and it's replaced with more oxygen. This process repeats itself over 100,000 times every day without any conscious thought on your part.

CHOLESTEROL

Contrary to what you may think, cholesterol is not all bad. You need cholesterol to make cell walls and hormones, but too much makes you more prone to heart disease. About 80 per cent of your cholesterol is manufactured by your liver and 20 per cent comes from the food you eat.

GOOD AND BAD CHOLESTEROL

Cholesterol is carried around the body in the blood by proteins called lipoproteins. Most of the cholesterol is carried by low-density lipoproteins, LDLs (which are mostly found in saturated fats), and it is these that are potentially harmful because they allow cholesterol to be deposited in the body. High-density lipoproteins, HDLs (found in poly- and monounsaturated fats), transport cholesterol back to the liver, thereby removing it from the blood and protecting your heart. So the aim is to keep your LDLs low and your HDLs high.

Get into the habit of looking at the fat content of foods and opt for foods that contain poly- or monounsaturated fats, which reduce your "bad" cholesterol. Other dietary measures you can take are described in the box (right).

▼ A daily diet that has at least five portions of fruit and vegetables can help maintain the health of your heart.

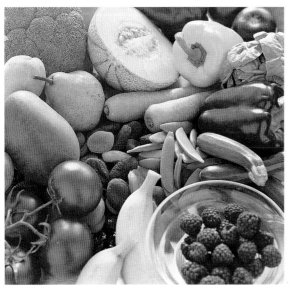

DR DAWN'S HEALTH CHECK
Diet for a healthy heart

There is no such thing as unhealthy food, just an unhealthy diet. A balanced diet should consist of:

• Carbohydrates – around half your daily calories should come from bread, cereals, and potatoes. Focus on wholegrain products, rather than refined carbohydrates such as white bread, pasta, and rice.

• Fruit and vegetables – aim for at least five portions a day. A glass of fruit juice counts as one portion (but only one, no matter how many you drink) and frozen fruit and vegetables can be just as nutritious as fresh. They are full of antioxidants to protect your heart.

• Milk and dairy products – are high in calcium, protein, and vitamins but opt for low-fat versions whenever possible. Aim for three portions a day.

• Meat and fish – provide iron, protein, vitamins, and minerals. Eat at least two portions of oily fish a week – mackerel, herring, sardine, and salmon (whether fresh, frozen, canned, or smoked) are all good sources of omega-3 fatty acids that protect against heart disease.

• Fats – a small amount of fat in your diet is essential as it provides vitamins A, D, E, and K as well as fatty acids, but high-fat diets can easily lead to obesity. You also need to watch the type of fat you are consuming – they can be subdivided into different types:

• Saturated fats – found in animal fats, full-fat dairy products, and products made with palm oil, such as biscuits, cakes, and pastries. These fats raise blood cholesterol levels and increase the risk of heart disease, and so your intake should be kept as low as possible.

• Trans fats – are even more harmful than saturated fats, and are created when vegetable oils are converted into hydrogenated fats. These fats increase bad cholesterol and decrease good cholesterol, increasing the risk of heart disease. They are commonly found in margarines, pastries, pies, biscuits, and cakes. Look at the ingredients of any foods that you buy, and avoid hydrogenated fat and partially hydrogenated fat.

• Monounsaturated fats – found in plant foods such as olive oil, nuts, and avocados. These lower bad cholesterol.

• Polyunsaturated fats – found in sunflower oil, some spreads, and oily fish. They also lower bad cholesterol, although not as effectively as monounsaturated fats.

SHOULD I BE WORRIED?

Blood cholesterol levels are measured in millimols of cholesterol per litre (mmol/l) of blood, and many people are confused about what their level of cholesterol should be. If you are worried about your level, ask your doctor for a test and they will be able to tell you if your results are within a healthy range. The number you should aim for will depend on different factors, including:

• Whether you are male or female.

• Your age.

• Your blood pressure.

If you are over 40, or have a family history of raised cholesterol, you should know your level, so ask your doctor for a test. For some people, high cholesterol means adjusting their diet, but as 80 per cent of your cholesterol is manufactured by your liver, for many it means taking medication, such as statins.

WHAT TO DO ABOUT HIGH CHOLESTEROL

The approach that you need to take will depend very much on your individual circumstances:

• If you are generally healthy, but have a raised cholesterol level, your first plan of action should be to make sure that you have a low-fat diet. Make sure that your intake of saturated fats is as low as possible, and replace them with unsaturated fats wherever you can. Your doctor should be able to provide you with nutritional information and advice to help you make the right food choices.

• Depending on your individual circumstances, your doctor may prescribe statins to decrease your blood cholesterol level. The higher your risk of coronary heart disease, the more likely it is that your doctor will recommend cholesterol-lowering drugs. However, statins will not be prescribed for everyone with high cholesterol. If you are in good health and have no other risk factors for coronary heart disease, your doctor may be happy for you to make lifestyle changes without taking medication.

FIND OUT MORE
www.bhf.org.uk

MYTH BUSTERS
Let's take a look at some of the myths surrounding cholesterol.

HAVING HIGH CHOLESTEROL MAKES ME MORE LIKELY TO HAVE A HEART ATTACK	TRUE	Although cholesterol is only one risk factor for developing coronary heart disease and taking action in other areas (such as stopping smoking, taking regular physical activity, controlling your weight and making sure your blood pressure is normal) are all essential to protecting against heart disease.
I ONLY EAT LOW-FAT FOOD, SO MY CHOLESTEROL LEVEL WILL BE LOW	FALSE	Only 20 per cent of your cholesterol level is determined by the food you eat, and the other 80 per cent is created by your liver. However, if you do have high cholesterol it is still important to follow a healthy diet (see the box on p.47).
CHOLESTEROL-LOWERING SPREADS DON'T WORK	FALSE	There are specific ranges of spreads, yoghurts, and milk products that have added plant sterols and stanols, and the evidence shows that they can help to reduce blood cholesterol levels. However, a healthy balanced diet is still important!

BLOOD PRESSURE

In the same way that you need pressure to push water through a garden hose, pressure is needed to pump blood around your body. The narrower the hosepipe, the higher the pressure needed to get the water on your garden; the same is true of the pressure in your arteries.

HOW IS BLOOD PRESSSURE MEASURED?

Blood pressure is given as two readings: the top (or first) number is called the systolic blood pressure and is the maximum pressure in the system; the bottom (or second) number is the diastolic blood pressure – the lowest pressure in the system.

WHAT ARE THE SYMPTOMS OF HIGH BLOOD PRESSURE?

Contrary to popular belief, most people with high blood pressure don't have any symptoms at all. While raised blood pressure can cause headaches and nosebleeds, this is the exception and not the norm. The best way to find out if you have high blood pressure is to have it checked by your doctor.

WHEN SHOULD YOU SEE A DOCTOR?

It is completely normal and appropriate for blood pressure to go up when we are in pain or frightened but if it is consistently high, then it puts a strain on your heart. Most doctors would want to retest blood pressure on several occasions before making a diagnosis of high blood pressure, known as hypertension.

If your blood pressure is consistently greater than 140/90 mmHg, you are hypertensive and you need to take measures to reduce it. If your blood pressure is only slightly raised, your doctor will suggest you adjust your lifestyle (see box right), but if it is consistently greater than 160/100 mmHg, you will probably have to take medication to bring it down.

Anyone over 40 should know their blood pressure and have it checked at least every five years. If it is borderline or you are on medication for raised blood pressure, your doctor will want to check it more frequently and will be able to tailor your treatment to your individual needs.

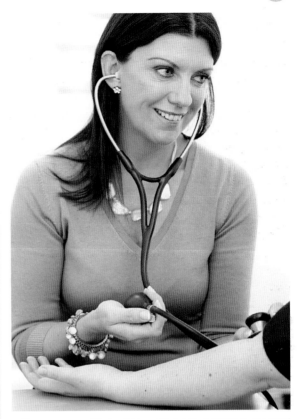

▲ *Everyone over 40 should have their blood pressure checked at least every five years.*

DR DAWN'S HEALTH CHECK
Bringing your blood pressure down without medication

- Lose any excess weight.
- If you smoke, then give up now.
- Stop adding salt to your food – it will taste bland at first but you will be amazed how quickly your taste buds adjust. After two to three weeks you will wonder how you managed to eat such salty food.
- Stick to a low-fat diet – fat should constitute less than 30 per cent of your total daily calorie intake, and of this, only a third should be saturated fat.
- Keep to the recommended daily limits for alcohol (see p.77).
- Take regular exercise – you should aim for 30 minutes at least five times week (see pp.54–55).
- Try to manage your stress.

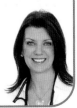

WHY IS BLOOD PRESSURE HIGHER AT THE DOCTOR'S SURGERY?

I often see people in surgery who tell me their home blood pressure monitor shows normal recordings but as soon as they come to the clinic the readings go up. This is a well-recognized phenomenon known as "white-coat hypertension". You may not feel anxious but subconsciously your sympathetic nervous system has kicked in – this is the part of your nervous system that you don't have conscious control of, but which is responsible for the reflex reaction of "fight or flight".

The first thing I do is to check the patient's own monitor against the one in surgery – if the home monitor correlates with mine, I know I can rely on the home readings. The jury is still out on how significant white-coat hypertension is, and what your doctor decides to do will depend on exactly what your readings are.

WHAT IS LOW BLOOD PRESSURE?

If your blood pressure is lower than 90/60 mmHg, then you will be considered to have low blood pressure.

Generally, doctors look to reduce blood pressure, and low blood pressure by itself does not necessarily cause

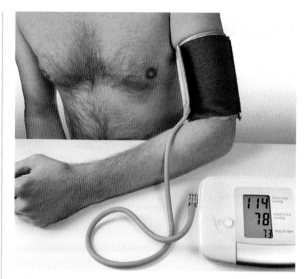

▲ Home monitors are a useful tool but make sure that you get them checked against your doctor's machine to make sure that they are accurate.

symptoms. However, if it gets too low then you run the risk of not getting enough blood to vital organs such as the brain and kidneys. Critically ill people in intensive care units often have dangerously low blood pressure and need powerful drugs given into the veins to support the heart.

Young women can be prone to low blood pressure. This isn't dangerous but can mean that if they stand still for long periods or stand up suddenly after sitting or lying they feel lightheaded and sometimes even faint. If you know your blood pressure is on the low side, simply drawing a circle in the air with your feet before you stand up and rocking back and forth on your heels when standing still should be enough to prevent dizzy spells. But remember, persistent dizzy episodes should be checked out by your doctor.

DR DAWN'S HEALTH CHECK
When do you need treatment?

Whether or not you need treatment depends on your overall risk of a heart attack or stroke, rather than simply on your blood pressure alone. To help evaluate this overall risk, doctors put people in two main categories:

Patients with no known coronary heart disease
• Blood pressure less than 140/90 – no treatment necessary.
• Blood pressure between 140/90 and 159/99 – treatment with lifestyle measures.
• Blood pressure 160/100 or over – treatment with medication.

Patients with coronary heart disease
• Diabetics with blood pressure 130/80 or over – treatment with medication.
• Non-diabetics with blood pressure 140/85 or over – treatment with medication.

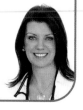

FIND OUT MORE
www.bpassoc.org.uk

ANGINA

This is the term we use to describe the pain that people feel when there is insufficient oxygen getting to the heart muscle. It is usually caused by furring up, or narrowing, of the blood vessels around the heart (the coronary arteries), so in fact the term "angina" refers to the symptoms of coronary heart disease and the two terms are pretty much interchangeable.

HOW WILL I RECOGNIZE IT?

The pain of angina is usually described as a heavy or crushing pain, as if someone is sitting on your chest. It may be central or left-sided, and it often radiates down the left arm and/or up towards the neck or jaw. The pain develops when your heart needs to work harder, for example during exercise, but it can be triggered by even modest increased demands on your heart, such as after a meal when blood is diverted to the gut to aid digestion. It is often associated with nausea, shortness of breath, and palpitations, and should never be ignored:

• It is important to rest if you develop these symptoms, and take any angina medication that you may have.

• If the symptoms do not subside within 20 minutes you should seek medical help urgently, as they will need investigation.

• Severe pain that doesn't ease when you rest or take your medication and continues for several minutes may be a heart attack. This should be treated as a medical emergency – dial 999.

> **! SEEK MEDICAL ADVICE NOW**
> **If you have chest pain that:**
> • Feels like a heavy weight on your chest.
> • Feels worse during exercise.
> • Radiates down towards your arm, or up towards your jaw.
> • Makes you short of breath.
> • Makes you sweaty.
> • Makes you feel sick.

HOW IS IT TREATED?

A diagnosis of angina is usually confirmed with a treadmill test, or a special X-ray of your blood vessels called an angiogram. You will then be prescribed medication to prevent attacks – you are likely to be prescribed a medication that you spray under your tongue when symptoms strike. It dilates the vessels around the heart, improving the circulation to the heart muscle. It's important to carry your medication with you at all times – it is no good to you in the bathroom cabinet at home! The aim will be to keep you symptom free, so if you continue to have angina attacks during treatment then you should see your doctor, as he or she may want to consider increasing your medication.

▾ Angina sprays are used to treat the condition, and are sprayed under the tongue when symptoms occur. However, it is important to carry the medication with you at all times.

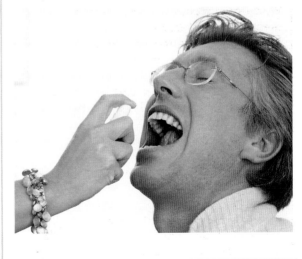

FIND OUT MORE
www.bhf.org.uk

CORONARY HEART DISEASE

Also called CHD, coronary artery disease, or ischaemic heart disease, this is the most common form of heart disease. Each year 300,000 people have heart attacks in the UK and more than 110,000 die as a result of heart problems. Not only is coronary heart disease the most common cause of premature death, it is also a major cause of disability and illness – around 1.5 million people in the UK suffer from angina.

WHAT IS CORONARY HEART DISEASE?

It is caused by narrowing, or hardening, of the arteries that supply blood to the heart muscle. Your doctor may also refer to it as either atheroma or atherosclerosis. The narrower the coronary arteries, the less well your heart is able to work. Think of your arteries as a three-lane motorway – if two lanes are coned off, the traffic slows down as it tries to filter into the single open lane. In exactly the same way, the blood in narrowed coronary arteries can not get to the heart muscle as quickly.

? DID YOU KNOW

Who is at risk

There are lots of different things that influence your risk of developing coronary heart disease. I like to classify the risk factors into things you can do nothing about and things you can avoid – the good news is there are lots more entries in the avoidable group!

Risk factors you can't avoid

• Being male, or female after the menopause.
• A family history of heart disease.
• Getting older.
• Diabetes – if it is unrelated to weight gain.

Risk factors you can avoid

• Smoking.
• Obesity.
• Diabetes – if it is related to weight gain.
• High blood pressure.
• High cholesterol.
• Lack of exercise.
• Stress.

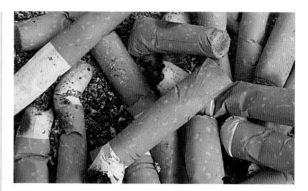

▲ Smoking puts you at a much higher risk of coronary heart disease, but it's never too late to give up.

When you exercise, your heart needs to work harder and it needs more oxygen. Healthy people can simply increase the amount of blood supplied to the muscle, but if you have coronary heart disease, the narrowed arteries just can't cope and you experience pain and/or shortness of breath – this is angina. If the arteries become completely blocked, no blood can get through to that part of the heart, and you suffer a heart attack, which could cause your heart to stop (cardiac arrest).

HOW YOU CAN AVOID RISK FACTORS

Over the last 30 years, deaths from coronary heart disease have fallen, but the UK death rate is still one of the highest in Western Europe. Perhaps most worrying is that death rates in young people are falling more slowly than in older people.

Smoking

Half of all smokers will eventually be killed by their habit, and you don't have to be a heavy smoker. One study of Danish women showed that smoking as few as three cigarettes a day could almost double the risk of death and heart attack. But it's never too late to give up. Just one year after quitting, the risk of developing heart disease is cut by half. After ten years, the risk of heart disease is the same as if you had never smoked.

FIND OUT MORE
www.givingupsmoking.co.uk

Obesity

Over the last two centuries, life expectancy has doubled in the Western world, but the trend is starting to reverse. Some experts now believe that we could be looking at a situation in which parents outlive their children. The main reason for this is obesity (see p.94). Britain is currently fattest nation in Europe, and we are rapidly catching up with America.

The number of children in Britain who are obese has tripled in the last 20 years: a boy who is seriously overweight as a child is 50 per cent more likely to die as a young man than if he was a normal weight. An obese woman is three times more likely to have a heart attack and 12 times more likely to develop diabetes; an obese man is one and half times more likely to have a heart attack and five times more likely to develop diabetes. (Interestingly, it's not just about how fat you are, but also where you carry your excess weight, see p.94.)

Diabetes

There are over two million people in the UK with diabetes. They are two to four times more likely to develop heart disease, and three-quarters of them will die of coronary heart disease.

High blood pressure

The higher your blood pressure, the greater your risk of developing heart disease and, contrary to popular belief, most people with high blood pressure don't get headaches or nosebleeds. Unless you have your blood pressure measured, there is no way of predicting what it is (see p.49).

Raised cholesterol

Nearly half of the 110,000 deaths from heart disease in the UK each year can be attributed at least in part to high cholesterol levels. It's estimated that a quarter of all men and women aged 16–24 have cholesterol levels above the recommended limits (see p.47). Unless you have a blood test, you cannot predict your blood cholesterol level. I think everyone over the age of 40 should know their blood cholesterol count and if you have heart disease in the family, you should get it checked before you are 40.

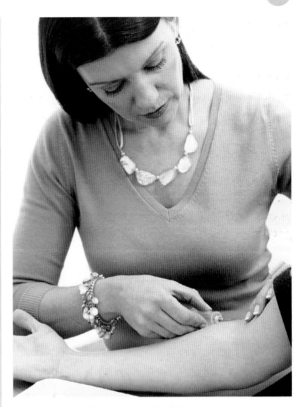

▲ *A blood test is the only way to find out your cholesterol level.*

Lack of exercise

Your heart is like any other muscle – if you don't use it, it will get out of condition. Every little helps, although ideally you should be exercising at least five times a week; push yourself so that your heart rate increases and you are puffing a bit – see pp.54–55.

Stress

This is very difficult to quantify – what winds one person up like a spinning top will waft straight over another person's head. A totally stress-free existence isn't possible and actually I don't think anyone would want it. A little stress can be stimulating, but working under constant pressure isn't good for you.

Try writing down all the things that hassle you and then take a long hard look at the list – there will be some things you either can't, or don't want to, alter but there will be others that with a little rearranging could be avoided.

WHAT SORT OF EXERCISE HELPS YOUR HEART?

The fitter you are, the less likely you are to develop heart problems. But there's more to it than that – people who exercise are also more likely to survive a heart attack if they have one.

The type of exercise that helps the heart the most is aerobic exercise. This is any repetitive activity involving the large muscles of the legs and/or arms. It doesn't have to involve high-tech gym equipment, just walking briskly, jogging, cycling, or dancing on a regular basis can be enough to make your heart work more efficiently. Even doing the vacuuming or other housework with some extra gusto will help.

According to the British Heart Foundation, only about one in three adults in the UK is exercising enough to protect themselves from developing coronary heart disease.

How much exercise?

Current guidelines suggest you should be exercising for 30 minutes at least five times a week. In addition, you should also aim to walk 10,000 paces a day. An average pace is 50–75cm (20–30in), so you would have to cover 5–7.5 km (3–4.5 miles) a day just going about your normal day-to-day business. A pedometer worn on your waistband will measure the number of steps you take. They are relatively cheap and they don't cheat. You might be horrified by how inactive you really are.

The most important thing to do when trying to increase your level of daily exercise is to choose something that you will enjoy – paying for gym membership may make you feel better, but unless you go regularly it may not be worth the money. For many people, incorporating more

---

DR DAWN'S HEALTH CHECK
Women and heart disease

If I asked you to describe a typical heart attack victim, you would no doubt describe a stressed, overweight, middle-aged man who takes no exercise and smokes. Of course you would be right, but heart disease is also the number one killer of women in the UK – five times as many women die from heart disease as from breast cancer.

The risk factors for CHD are the same for women as they are for men but the weighting can be different:

• Smoking – smoking carries almost twice the risk of heart disease in women than in men.

• Obesity – about one-third of women in the UK are overweight and one in five are clinically obese.

• Diabetes – women with diabetes have a three-fold increased risk of developing coronary heart disease compared to those without the disease, and a woman with diabetes who has a heart attack is eight times more likely to die as a result than a woman without it.

• High blood pressure – a woman with hypertension has a 3.5 times greater risk of developing heart disease than a woman without hypertension.

• High cholesterol – before the menopause women's oestrogen levels have a natural protective effect against high cholesterol, but after the menopause cholesterol levels are likely to rise.

• Exercise – women seem to give up formal exercise earlier than men. According to the British Heart Foundation, two-thirds of British women are so unfit that they cannot walk at a normal pace up a gradual slope without becoming breathless.

• Stress – more women are juggling the pressures of work and home. My guess is we are generally more stressed than our grandmothers were.

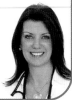

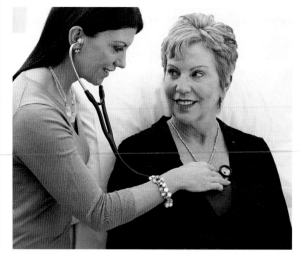

▾ *Heart disease is the biggest killer of women in the UK, so it's important to look after your heart.*

exercise into daily life is more successful – think about cycling to work, or if this is not practical, park your car a little way away and walk the rest. Take the stairs, rather than lifts or escalators. Walk to the shops instead of taking the bus. Incorporating more activity into your life really will make a difference. However, if you are not used to exercising, don't take up a strenuous activity without talking to your doctor first – start slowly.

How do you know if you are exercising hard enough?

The "talk test" is a simple way of judging how hard you are working. If you can talk easily while you are exercising, you aren't pushing yourself enough; if you are gasping and unable to talk at all, you should slow down. Somewhere in the middle is just right. If you are taking up exercise from having been a bit of a couch potato, remember to increase your levels of activity gradually – to begin with, it won't take much to get you out of breath.

Measure your pulse

If you are serious about getting your heart in shape, it's worth investing in a pulse monitor. These are worn on your wrist like a watch, or as a band around your chest, and it will tell you how hard your heart is working. During exercise you should aim for a pulse rate that is about 70–85 per cent of your maximum heart rate (MHR), although if you are new to exercise you should start off by aiming for 60 per cent of your MHR and increase the intensity of your exercise slowly.

To calculate your MHR, subtract your age from 220, so for example, if you are 40, your MHR will be 180, making your optimum training range 70–85 per cent of 180 (about 126–153 beats per minute).

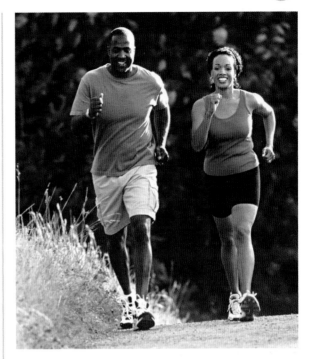

▲ You should aim to exercise five times a week for at least 30 minutes.

WHAT ELSE CAN I DO?

Although exercise is essential to a healthy heart, it is also important to make other lifestyle changes to reduce your risk of coronary heart disease:

● Give up smoking (see pp.70–71 for advice on how to kick the habit).

● Reduce your blood pressure (see p.48 for some positive changes you can make to reduce your blood pressure).

● Eat a healthy balanced diet (see the box on p.47 for advice on what you should be eating).

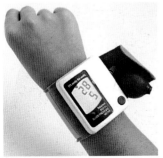

◄ It can be worth investing in a pulse rate monitor if you exercise regularly.

FIND OUT MORE
www.bhf.org.uk

HEART ATTACK

A heart attack is caused by a blockage of the blood supply to part of the heart muscle. The main risk is that it will cause the heart to stop suddenly – this is called a cardiac arrest and is an absolute medical emergency. Around 70 per cent of all cardiac arrests in the UK occur outside of the hospital environment and knowing what to do really could save a life.

WHAT HAPPENS IN A CARDIAC ARREST?

During a cardiac arrest the heart stops pumping and the brain and other organs no longer receive a supply of oxygenated blood. The first three minutes of a cardiac arrest are crucial, as after this time brain damage will occur; and after five minutes, the person is likely to die unless they are given cardiac massage (see box right).

WHAT SHOULD YOU DO?

If you suspect that someone is having a heart attack, then you should dial 999 immediately. Ask for an ambulance and tell the control officer you think it is a heart attack. He or she will talk you through what you need to do while you are waiting for the paramedics to arrive. The steps that you should take to resuscitate someone are shown on the right.

WHAT IS THE MEDICAL TREATMENT?

Paramedics will conduct an electrocardiography (ECG) to check the heart rhythm and will treat it appropriately – either by administering an electric shock using an electric defibrillator, or by injecting adrenaline to start the heart again.

FIND OUT MORE
www.sja.org.uk

! EMERGENCY – DIAL 999
What to do if someone has a heart attack

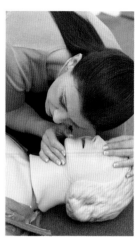

1 Check if person is unconscious – tap his or her shoulder and call out the name. If there is no response, the person is unconscious.

Tilt the head back to open the air passages. Check if the person is breathing – place your cheek by his or her mouth, look along the chest and listen and feel for air coming from the mouth and nose. If you can't see or feel anything, the person is not breathing. Call for help – get someone to call an ambulance. If you are in a public place, ask for a defibrillator (a special machine that may be able to restart the heart).

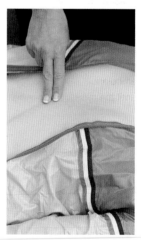

2 Prepare to start chest compressions by finding the place to press down on the chest. Find one of the lowermost ribs using the first two fingers of the hand closest to the person's legs. Slide your fingers along the rib to the point where the lowermost ribs meet the breastbone. Place your middle finger here and your index finger above it on the lower breastbone. Put the heel of your other hand on the breastbone and slide it down until it reaches your index finger. This is where you should press to give chest compressions.

3 Start chest compressions. Place one hand on the centre of the person's chest. Cover this with your other hand. Leaning right over the person's chest with your arms vertical and straight, press down on the chest. Then release the pressure but don't remove your hands – this is a chest compression. Repeat this 30 times at a rate of 100 per minute.

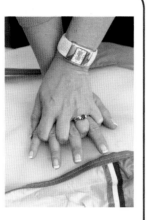

4 Move to the person's head. Tilt it back, lift the chin with one hand - this should open the mouth. Pinch the nose closed, take a breath, place your mouth over the person's mouth, and blow until the chest rises. Repeat this. Continue giving 30 chest compressions followed by two breaths of mouth-to-mouth until the ambulance arrives. If you are alone, give compressions and mouth-to-mouth for one minute then call an ambulance. Resume compressions and mouth-to-mouth until the ambulance arrives.

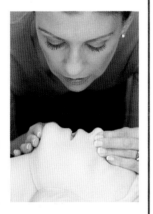

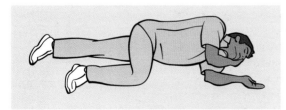

5 If the person is unconscious but breathing, place him or her on to the side with head tilted back. The upper arm and leg should be at right angles to the body to prevent him or her rolling forward. This is called the recovery position and keeps the airways open.

AFTER A HEART ATTACK

A heart attack is a major event, both physically and emotionally, and it will take time to recover. Initially, you will be in hospital and will have a lot of information to take on board while you are there. Your main focus will be getting through each day and becoming well enough to go home. In my experience, it's only when you are back at home that the reality sinks in and you start to ask questions – here are some of the most common ones that I am asked.

WHEN CAN I RETURN TO WORK?

It is estimated that nearly 2 million working days are lost each year because of vascular disease, which includes heart disease and strokes.

For many patients, returning to work is a crucial part of regaining their self-esteem and confidence, but how quickly that can happen depends both on the type of work involved and your attitude to it. Traditionally, cardiologists have reviewed heart attack patients two months or so after the event, before giving the all-clear to return to work, and in most cases this seems sensible. In fact, delaying the return to work for more than three months can make a successful return less likely as prolonged periods away from work can leave us lacking in confidence to return, regardless of why we are off. The exception to this rule is people who have had bypass surgery (an operation to bypass the blocked artery), who may need six months to recover.

WHEN CAN I START DRIVING AGAIN?

The DVLA will allow you to drive four weeks after a heart attack provided you have your doctor's agreement.

WHEN IS IT SAFE TO FLY?

It is sensible to delay flying for at least three weeks after a heart attack.

WHEN CAN I HAVE SEX AGAIN?

I once worked with a cardiologist who had a stock answer to this question: "three weeks with the wife, six weeks with the mistress". Joking apart, provided there are no complications it is perfectly safe to resume your sex life two to three weeks after a heart attack.

WHEN CAN I START EXERCISING AGAIN?

Most people who have been hospitalized because of a heart problem will be offered a comprehensive rehabilitation programme where their individual concerns will be addressed. These usually start six weeks after a heart attack.

It is vital that you listen to your body after a heart attack. How much exercise you can do will depend a bit on your age and how fit you were before. The important thing is not to ignore discomfort or pain.

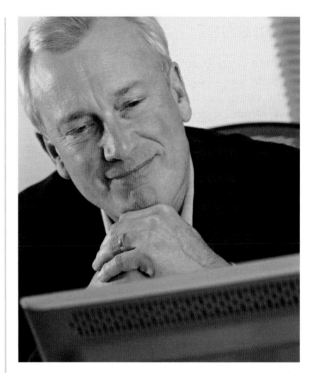

▲ *Returning to work after a heart attack can be a positive step on the road to recovery.*

FIND OUT MORE
www.cardiacrehabilitation.org.uk

MYTH BUSTERS
Let's take a look at some of the myths surrounding heart disease.

HEART DISEASE MAINLY AFFECTS MIDDLE-AGED MEN WHO DON'T GET ENOUGH EXERCISE	FALSE	Heart disease is actually the number one killer of women in the UK, and the risk factors for men and women are the same.
NOW THAT I HAVE HAD A HEART ATTACK, IT'S ONLY A MATTER OF TIME BEFORE I HAVE ANOTHER	FALSE	Even after you have had a heart attack you can make positive lifestyle changes that will put you in a lower risk category, for example by stopping smoking, eating healthily, and exercising.
HEART DISEASE RUNS IN MY FAMILY SO I AM MUCH MORE LIKELY TO HAVE A HEART ATTACK	TRUE	If any members of your immediate family (mother, father, brother, or sister) have suffered coronary heart disease or angina at a young age (under 65 for women and under 55 for men), you could be at increased risk of developing coronary heart disease – speak to your doctor.
TAKING THE CONTRACEPTIVE PILL FOR A LONG TIME INCREASES THE RISK OF A HEART ATTACK	TRUE	But in most healthy women, with no other heart disease factors, the risk is still lower than the risks associated with pregnancy.

VARICOSE VEINS

Arteries carry blood away from the heart to all parts of the body and the blood returns in the veins. Unlike arteries, veins do not have elastic walls and they rely on one-way valves at regular intervals to prevent the blood slipping backwards. If these valves are under too much pressure, they start to fail and leak, which is what causes the dilated blue veins we know as varicose veins.

WHO IS AT RISK?

Anyone can get varicose veins. In general, women are more prone to them than men but those most at risk are:
- Pregnant women. Pregnancy raises the pressure in the veins, making varicose veins much more likely.
- Those with a family history of varicose veins.
- People who stand for long periods – I have lots of hairdressers who are plagued by varicose veins.
- Being obese – although only if you are a woman.
- Smoking – there is some controversy among specialists about this, but as far as I am concerned, it certainly won't help.

WHAT YOUR DOCTOR MAY ADVISE?

Once the valves have been damaged and are starting to leak, the only thing that really works is an operation to remove the damaged vein. Whether or not you decide to go down that route depends on how much they bother you – varicose veins can cause tired, aching legs. If they are just a bit unsightly, you can consider having them injected (called sclerotherapy). This process involves injecting a chemical directly into the vein to close it completely, and works best on smaller veins. This is usually done as an outpatient procedure by a vascular surgeon and takes about 30 minutes. You won't need a general anaesthetic and you can go straight back to work afterwards. However, be prepared to make more than one trip – you will need two sessions if just one leg is affected and at least three if it is both.

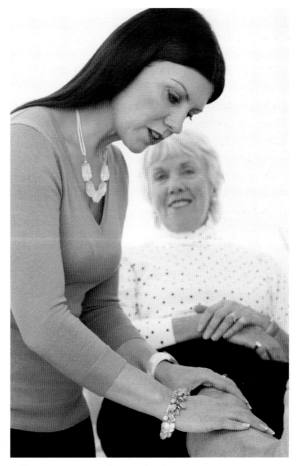

▲ Anyone can get varicose veins, but women are more prone to them than men.

DR DAWN'S HEALTH CHECK
Preventing varicose veins

Like all things, prevention is better than cure, and if you are concerned about varicose veins you should:
- Keep active. If your work means you have to stand up for long periods, fidget! Just rocking back and forward on your heels will get the calf muscle pumping and help keep blood flowing back to the heart.
- Lose weight if you are carrying excess pounds.
- If you smoke, give up now.
- Wear support tights.
- Consider taking red vine leaf extract, which is a herbal remedy that promotes healthy veins and capillaries.

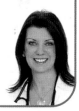

DEEP VEIN THROMBOSIS

A deep vein thrombosis (DVT) is a blood clot that forms in the deep veins of the leg, making the leg hot, red, swollen, and painful. The main concern is that part of the clot could break off and travel around the circulatory system to the lung. There it could form something called a pulmonary embolism that could block the major blood vessel supplying the lungs, and can be fatal.

WHO IS AT RISK?

Anything that makes the blood more likely to clot in the veins will put you at risk of a DVT. Common risk factors include:

- Immobility – especially if in bed for any length of time, say because of illness or after an operation.
- Long-haul air travel (see Holidays and travel health, p.205).
- Pregnancy.
- Obesity.
- Smoking.
- Taking the combined contraceptive pill.
- Increasing age.
- A family history of deep vein thrombosis – some families pass on a genetic tendency to blood clots. If you have a first-degree relative (that is, mother, father, or sibling) who developed a DVT out of the blue without any obvious cause, you should talk to your doctor about having a blood test to check out something called thrombophilia.
- Varicose veins – but these have to be severe. The odd blue vein on the back of your leg won't give you a DVT.

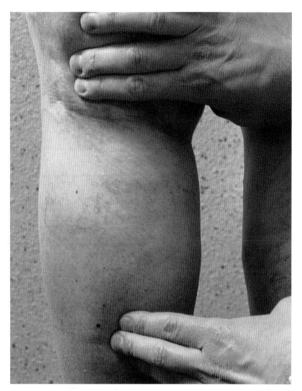

▲ Deep vein thrombosis can cause painful swelling in the leg.

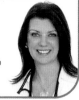

DR DAWN'S HEALTH CHECK
How can I prevent DVT?

Sadly, you can't change advancing years or genetics, but you can minimize your risks by:

- Keeping active.
- Stopping smoking.
- Losing excess weight.
- Considering an alternative to the combined contraceptive pill – there are lots available. However, don't stop taking your pill before considering alternative contraception.
- During a long flight, get up and walk around once an hour. Wearing compression tights can also help. If you are driving for a long time make sure that you stop regularly to have a short walk.
- At times of imposed immobility, such as being in bed after an operation, stretch your legs if possible. Your doctor may also recommend compression stockings.

! SEEK MEDICAL ADVICE NOW
If you experience the following:

- Suden onset of pain in the calf or thigh.
- One calf swelling to 3cm greater that the other calf.
- Newly swollen veins in a painful limb.

PALPITATIONS

When most people talk about palpitations they are talking about the feeling that their heart is racing or fluttering in their chest. Everyone experiences this at some time – waiting to go into an exam or to a big interview can give all but the most confident of us palpitations.

ARE THEY SERIOUS?

Apart from being caused by anxiety, you may feel heart palpitations after a big meal or after exercising, but how do you know when palpitations indicate a more serious problem? If you know you are nervous or you have just pushed yourself physically, the chances are you have nothing to worry about. However, if you are experiencing palpitations without a reason you should see your doctor.

DR DAWN'S HEALTH CHECK
Managing your palpitations

If you suffer from palpitations and you have had your heart checked, the following tips may help you control them:

• Manage your stress – keeping a diary of when your palpitations occur can help you identify a pattern, which might suggest changes to help.
• Cut out caffeine, which is in coffee, tea, and cola.
• Watch your alcohol intake – drinking excessively can cause palpitations.
• Stop smoking – nicotine is a stimulant.
• Some decongestants can cause palpitations but never stop any prescribed medication without your doctor's advice.

! SEEK MEDICAL ADVICE NOW
If, when you have palpitations, you:

• Feel an irregular heartbeat.
• Are resting and not knowingly anxious.
• Have chest pain, feel lightheaded, or faint.
• Feel nauseous, clammy, or sweaty.
• Are short of breath.

Most will be harmless, but it's better to be safe than sorry.

ANAEMIA

Oxygen is carried from the lungs to all parts of our body in red blood cells (on haemoglobin molecules), which also carry carbon dioxide back to the lungs. We measure haemoglobin (Hb) in grams per deciliter (g/dl) and normal values of Hb are 13.5–18 g/dl for men, and 11.5–16 g/dl for women. Women tend to have lower haemoglobin levels, not least because they lose blood every month during menstruation.

WHAT CAUSES IT?

If your blood haemoglobin level falls below normal this is called anaemia. The most common cause of this is an iron deficiency. Iron is found in the diet in liver, green leafy vegetables, pulses, meat, and some seafood.

Being low in vitamin B12 or folate can also cause anaemia, as can being pregnant, taking certain drugs, or having other illnesses, such as chronic kidney disease, thyroid problems, and some arthritic conditions. To make sure you absorb dietary iron efficiently, eat iron-rich foods on an empty stomach with a fruit juice rich in vitamin C.

WHAT ARE THE SYMPTOMS?

I think of anaemia as trying to function on half a tank of fuel. Symptoms include:

• Lack of energy.
• Shortness of breath on mild exertion, or even at rest in extreme cases.
• Looking very pale.
• Palpitations, and even chest pain.

SHOULD I SEE A DOCTOR?

Anaemia can be caused by dietary iron deficiency but there are other conditions that cause it. You really need to know what is causing your particular anaemia to know how to treat it, and just taking iron supplements or multivitamins may not improve your symptoms. If you think you could be anaemic, you need to see your doctor or practice nurse for a blood test to confirm the diagnosis. If you are anaemic, your doctor will want to look into why and then tailor treatment to your specific needs.

• You breathe in at least 10,000 litres (17,500 pints) of air every day through your lungs • The surface area of the air sacs (alveoli) is so great that if smoothed out flat they would cover the entire surface of a tennis court • Your respiratory system produces about 2.2 litres (4 pints) of thin mucus every day without you even knowing • Even an individual with a sedentary lifestyle will take around 400 million breaths in an average lifetime.

5
Respiratory system

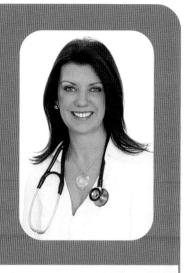

Introduction Our lungs never rest. When you breathe in, air containing oxygen enters the body through your mouth and nose, and then passes down a large tube called the trachea. At its base this tube divides into two smaller tubes (bronchi) – one for each lung. These tubes divide again hundreds of times into smaller and smaller tubes, each ending in one of hundreds of millions of air sacs (alveoli) that look like microscopic raspberries. Once in the lung, oxygen passes to the blood and at the same time carbon dioxide, the waste product of breathing, is removed from the blood to be breathed out. Muscles around the airways and the chest, and the large, flat sheet of muscle under the lungs called the diaphragm, help the lungs expand during breathing.

Air is warmed (or cooled) and moistened as it passes down the airways to the alveolar sacs. Tiny hairs, called cilia, also trap particles of dirt and other debris, preventing them from reaching the lungs. All this happens night and day without you having to do anything.

ASTHMA

There are over five million people in the UK with asthma. This is a long-term condition that can cause the muscles surrounding the walls of the airways to contract, making them smaller, and inflame the lining of the airways, both of which make breathing more difficult. This is normally triggered by contact with an allergen.

WHO DOES IT AFFECT?

Most people know someone with asthma. Not only does it vary in intensity from person to person, most asthmatics will also tell you they go through phases when their asthma doesn't bother them at all, and other times when they really struggle. It is known that having a close relative with asthma puts you at risk of developing the condition, but what triggers a flare-up for you could be completely different to theirs.

WHAT TRIGGERS AN ASTHMA ATTACK?

There are many different triggers; common ones include:

• Exercise.

• Allergens, such as pollen or animal fur.

• Cigarette smoke.

• Damp weather.

• Upper respiratory tract infections.

• Stress.

• Some medications, such as ibuprofen or aspirin.

WHAT YOUR DOCTOR WILL ADVISE

Most asthmatics manage their condition with inhalers and there are two main types – "relievers" (usually blue) that open up the airways and are used when breathing is difficult, and steroid-based "preventers" (usually brown or white) that reduce inflammation and which are generally used daily.

Young children may find using an inhaler difficult to coordinate – your doctor will be able to provide a spacer device to make things easier. You may also be given a peak flow meter to monitor your asthma at home. Most practices hold asthma clinics run by a practice nurse where your asthma can be regularly monitored. People with more severe asthma may need to take tablets and use nebulizers at home.

? DID YOU KNOW

Living with asthma

In my experience, many asthmatics put up with less than perfect breathing, believing that is the nature of their condition. The Royal College of Physicians has devised three simple questions for you to ask yourself:

• Have you had difficulty sleeping because of your asthma symptoms?

• Have you experienced coughing, wheezing, chest tightness, or breathlessness during the day?

• Does your asthma interfere with your usual activities, such as housework, work, school, sport, and so on?

If the answer to any of the questions is yes, talk to your doctor – your treatment probably could be improved.

! FIRST AID FOR AN ATTACK

Give a blue inhaler – it should start to work within three minutes, but if it doesn't then give another dose. If the inhaler does not work after five minutes and the person seems to be worsening (especially if their breathlessness is making talking difficult), then call an ambulance immediately.

FIND OUT MORE
www.asthma.org.uk

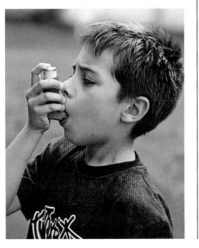

Blue inhalers (relievers) are used to open the airways when breathing feels difficult. ▶

COMMON COLD

This is a common viral infection that causes inflammation of the lining of your nose and throat, giving you a runny or blocked nose, headache, and possibly a cough. Most colds clear up within a week or so. There is very little you can do if you catch a cold (and you can expect two or three a year), although you can reduce your risk of getting one.

REDUCING THE RISK

Healthy eating is a good place to start. Doctors don't talk about eating five portions of fruit and vegetables a day for nothing: they are packed with vitamin C and other antioxidants that will boost your immune system. If you smoke you will absorb only 70 per cent of your dietary vitamin C, so consider taking a supplement.

Washing your hands can help prevent the spread, as most colds are passed on by hand-to-hand contact, and from there to your eyes and nose.

WHAT YOU CAN DO IF YOU HAVE A COLD

Taking the herbal remedy echinacea may reduce the duration of the symptoms, so is worth a try, but if you are taking any other medicines do check with your doctor first. Echinacea can cause liver problems, and if taken in combination with drugs that affect the liver it could be harmful. High-dose vitamin C (500mg twice a day) and zinc may also reduce the duration of cold symptoms.

▾ *Vitamin C can help to boost your immune system.*

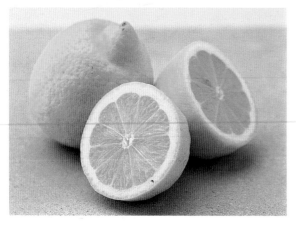

CATARRH

We all produce mucus from cells lining our nose and sinuses (spaces in the skull around the nose) and it's essential that we do – the mucus helps to trap bacteria and viruses, which are then swallowed into the gut and excreted rather than allowed into the airways where they could cause infection. Problems arise when we produce too much, or the mucus becomes thicker.

WHAT CAUSES IT?

Excessively thick mucus is often linked to central heating or bacterial infection, whereas the production of large volumes of thinner mucus is more likely to be caused by an allergy or viral infection. It can even be caused by some medicines, including the contraceptive pill.

WHAT YOU CAN DO

Treating catarrh can be notoriously difficult. People often resort to decongestants, which can help in the short term but your body becomes used to them and you can end up with worse problems when you stop them if you take them for more than a few days. A good old-fashioned steam inhalation with menthol is worth a try if you have catarrh due to a cold. If you think you may have an allergy, talk to your doctor as a course of antihistamines or a nasal spray may help.

CAN DAIRY PRODUCTS MAKE CATARRH WORSE?

Some people find dairy products make it worse. If you think that this is the case, then try cutting out dairy products for a few weeks. If your symptoms improve, reintroduce dairy just to make sure this isn't coincidental. If the catarrh comes back with a vengeance, it may be worth cutting dairy out long term. However, make sure you talk to a dietitian or your doctor because you must replace the nutrients dairy products provide.

INFLUENZA

This virus, commonly known as flu, is unique in that it changes each year, which is why last year's vaccine won't protect you from this year's strain. Most people recover from flu within a week or two.

WHAT ARE THE SYMPTOMS OF FLU?

Flu is far more debilitating than a cold – the symptoms develop over 24–48 hours and are much more severe. A friend of mine always says that if someone drops a winning lottery ticket on your doorstep when you have a cold, you will drag yourself out of your sickbed to pick it up; but if you have flu, you just can't be bothered or won't be able to get out of bed. That's probably an accurate reflection of just how terrible you feel with flu – you only have to have it once to never want it again. Typical symptoms include:

- Sudden onset of a high fever.
- Exhaustion.
- Dry cough.
- Headache.
- Aching muscles and joints.
- Sore throat.

It can also be normal to experience fatigue even after the other symptoms have gone.

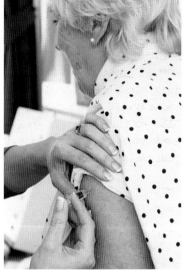

Flu vaccinations are free for everyone over 65. ▸

WHAT YOU CAN DO

The symptoms of flu can come on very quickly and the only thing you will want to do is go to bed. Make sure you have plenty of fluids, and regular paracetamol and/or ibuprofen to reduce the fever.

CAN THE VACCINE GIVE YOU FLU?

No. There is no live virus in the injection so you can't catch flu from having the jab. Every year I meet people who are convinced they contracted it from the vaccine, but they didn't; they must have been incubating it at the time of vaccination.

DR DAWN'S HEALTH CHECK
Have the flu vaccine

Flu is much more serious for the elderly or for those with a weakened immune system, as they are more likely to need hospital admission. You are eligible for free flu vaccines if you:

- Are over 65.
- Have diabetes.
- Have chronic heart disease.
- Have chronic lung disease.
- Have chronic kidney disease.
- Have a compromised immune system.
- Live hall accommodation.

If you don't fall into any of these groups, it is well worth considering having the vaccination privately.

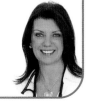

? DID YOU KNOW
Bird flu

Bird flu is a highly infectious disease amongst birds. There are many different strains, but the one that has hit the headlines is the deadly strain H5N1. It is only caught by very close contact with infected birds.

Symptoms in humans develop 3–5 days after infection and include a high fever, aching muscles, diarrhoea, sore throat, cough, and shortness of breath. The current flu vaccination won't protect against it, but since the arrival of bird flu in the UK, poultry workers are being offered a vaccination. This will eradicate the risk of bird flu mutating to a form that can be passed between humans.

PNEUMONIA

Pneumonia is inflammation of the lungs. It is usually due to infection, although it can also be caused by inhaling vomit, smoke, or chemicals. It affects as many as one in 100 of us each year and can strike at any age, but is most common in the elderly. The symptoms usually develop quickly and include cough, fever, difficult or painful breathing, and fatigue.

WHAT IS THE DIFFERENCE BETWEEN A CHEST INFECTION AND PNEUMONIA?

A chest infection can be an infection anywhere in the chest. It can sometimes be used to describe pneumonia (infection in the lung tissue) and other times to mean bronchitis (infection in the airways leading to the lung tissue). "Double pneumonia" means that both the lungs are involved.

WHO IS AT RISK?

- The very young (under 2) or those over 65.
- Smokers, heavy drinkers, and intravenous drug users.
- People with underlying respiratory problems, such as asthma, or coronary obstructive pulmonary disease.
- Anyone who has had an infection such as influenza.
- Those with a weakened immune system, for example, from chemotherapy or HIV infection.
- People who have had their spleen removed.

HOW IS PNEUMONIA DIAGNOSED?

Most cases of pneumonia are diagnosed by a physical examination of your chest, but your doctor may want to arrange a chest X-ray to confirm the extent of the inflammation, and may ask you for a sample of your sputum so that it can be analyzed to identify the exact cause of your infection.

PROTECTING YOURSELF

Anyone at risk should have an annual flu jab, and should talk to their doctor about having a pneumococcal vaccine. Pneumococcus is the commonest cause of bacterial pneumonia and, unlike the flu jab, most of us will only need one vaccination in a lifetime.

HAYFEVER

Also called allergic rhinitis, this is inflammation of the lining of the nose and throat caused by an allergy to pollen. Of course, it does not cause a fever and often has nothing to do with hay! Hayfever usually develops in the late teens but it can start earlier.

WHAT ARE THE SYMPTOMS?

The symptoms of itching and runny eyes and nose are due to the allergy, and the timing of your symptoms gives a clue to your specific allergy. If you develop symptoms in March or April you are probably reacting to silver birch, London plane, ash, or willow. Symptoms of grass pollen allergy (timothy, rye, and fescue) come on from May to July, and weed pollens (dock, nettle, or plantain) and mould spores cause trouble in July and August.

The number of people suffering from hayfever has quadrupled in the last 30 years, but no one really knows why. One possible theory is the effect of global warming on the life cycle of trees and grasses.

▾ *Wind dispersal of pollen can lead to a high pollen index, especially on warm, sunny days.*

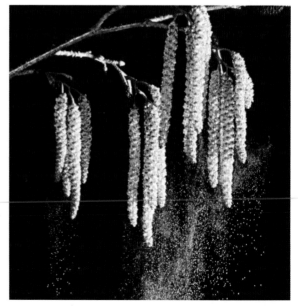

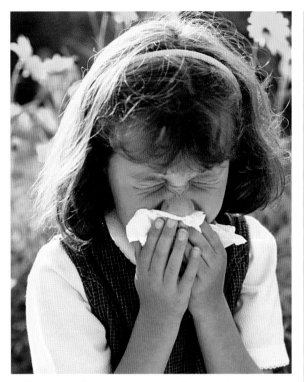

▲ *The timing of hayfever symptoms will give a clue to the specific pollen to which you are allergic.*

YOU CAN PREDICT THE POLLEN LEVELS

The presence of pollen is given as a pollen count – weather forecasters often give a pollen index in their reports when it's high. As a general rule, pollen counts are highest on sunny days when there is a stable, high-pressure weather system. They tend to dip first thing in the morning, then rise as the dew evaporates. When the air heats during the middle of the day, the pollens rise into the upper atmosphere and the count can fall but it increases again later, peaking in the early evening as the air cools again. Peak counts occur earlier in the evening in rural areas than in cities, where the air remains warmer for longer. Contrary to popular belief, hayfever tends to be more of a problem in urban areas than it is in the country. That may sound illogical given that there are fewer plants in cities, but it's probably due to the additive effect of traffic fumes and pollens.

WHAT YOU CAN DO

Treatment depends very much on severity of symptoms. You can manage mild symptoms by simply staying indoors when the count is very high, keeping windows and doors shut. Wear wraparound sunglasses if you go out, and buy a car fitted with a pollen filter.

Eye drops and nasal sprays help runny eyes and noses, but many people take antihistamine tablets, available from your chemist. Talk to your pharmacist about which one is best for you – the older types tend to cause drowsiness (no bad thing if you are struggling to sleep at night, but not ideal if you need to be alert for work); some of the newer ones are less sedating.

A recent study published in the *British Medical Journal* showed that the herbal remedy butterbur was as effective as traditional antihistamines for hayfever. I have suggested this to lots of my patients with some great results and, unlike some antihistamines, it doesn't cause any drowsiness.

WHAT ABOUT STEROIDS?

I reserve oral steroids for the most severe cases. I am often asked about steroid injections too. Doctors used to use them a lot and they worked very well, but the doses needed and the fact that they need to be repeated annually greatly increases your risk of osteoporosis (brittle-bone disease, see p.116) later in life so they are not recommended. If you can't control your symptoms, talk to your doctor about referral for immunotherapy.

> **?** **DID YOU KNOW**
> ### House dust mites
> Runny eyes or noses that persist all year round are unlikely to be due to pollens, so what else could it be? House dust mites are one of the most common causes of allergy. Sadly, you will never rid yourself of them completely, but you can reduce their numbers significantly by taking some important measures around the home:
> • Wash curtains, rugs, and bed linen regularly.
> • Soft toys are a good breeding ground for the mites – wash them weekly and then place them in a bag in the freezer for 24 hours.
> • Considering using hypoallergenic bed linen and pillows.
> • Wipe dust off floor surfaces daily, and off other surfaces regularly.
> • Vacuum carpets regularly.

SMOKING

Did you know that there are more than 4,000 different toxins in cigarette smoke? Smoking-related problems kill around 2,500 people every week in the UK and costs the NHS nearly £2 billion a year. Smokers make up 28 per cent of British men and 24 per cent of women – if you are one of them, read on; I have some frightening statistics.

SMOKING FACTS AND FIGURES

• Half of all smokers will die as a result of smoking-related diseases.

• A third of fire deaths in people over 70 are thought to be due to smoking.

• If you smoke, your children are three times more likely to smoke.

• 450 kids start smoking every day.

• Smoking when pregnant increases the risk of still birth, premature birth, and cot death.

• In the UK, out of every 1,000 young people who smoke 20 or more cigarettes a day, one will be murdered, six will die in road accidents, and 500 will die of smoking-related diseases.

PASSIVE SMOKING

Tobacco smoke is made up of the smoke that we inhale and "sidestream smoke" that comes from the burning tip of a cigarette. Since sidestream smoke hasn't passed through a filter it has a higher concentration of toxins than inhaled smoke. In a smoky atmosphere, 85 per cent of the smoke is sidestream smoke.

Nonsmokers who are exposed to passive smoking at home have a 25 per cent greater risk of developing lung cancer and heart disease (without ever smoking). If you smoke, your children are exposed to the equivalent of them smoking 60–150 cigarettes a year, and they are:

• Twice as likely to have asthma and chest infections.

• More likely to die of cot death.

• More at risk of meningitis.

• Be off school with coughs and colds more often.

• More likely to need hospital admission within their first year of life.

MYTH BUSTERS
Let's take a look at some of the myths that we hear about smoking.

I ONLY SMOKE LOW-TAR CIGARETTES SO I AM LESS AT RISK	FALSE	Smokers of low-tar cigarettes actually take in higher levels of tar and nicotine than suggested by the packaging because they draw harder to get the nicotine they crave.
IT IS NORMAL TO HAVE A COUGH IN THE MORNING IF YOU ARE A SMOKER	FALSE	If you smoke and have a cough in the morning, you probably already have irreversible lung damage.
MY CHILDREN ARE NOT AT RISK BECAUSE I DON'T SMOKE WHEN THEY ARE IN THE ROOM	FALSE	It takes about two hours for the smoke from a single cigarette to clear an average room. If you can't give up, at least smoke outside your house.
THE OCCASIONAL CIGARETTE WHEN PREGNANT WON'T DO ANY HARM	FALSE	Every time you smoke a cigarette while you are pregnant, the blood flow to your baby is reduced for 15 minutes. This causes the baby to be distressed and its heart rate increases to compensate.

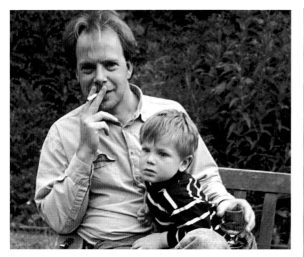

▲ *If you smoke, your children are three times more likely to become smokers when they are older.*

GIVING UP SMOKING

This isn't easy – no one ever said it was – but there are certainly more options available to help smokers now than ever before. If you are serious about giving up, here are a few tips to get you started:

• Work out what you spend on cigarettes in a week, a month, and a year, and how much you would save.

• Make a list of the reasons you want to smoke and the reasons you want to stop – which is the longer?

• Keep a diary of when you smoke to help you identify triggers like being on a coffee break. Recognizing your weak points will give you a better chance of avoiding temptation in the days ahead.

• Set a date to quit. You will need to be feeling strong – if you are under a lot of pressure, now may not be the best time, but don't look for excuses.

• Make a plan for what you will do instead – taking up a new hobby may help take your mind off things.

• Think about how you will cope when you have weak moments – one patient of mine promised herself she could have a cigarette if she still wanted it in 10 minutes and then took herself off for a shower. A walk round the block could also be helpful. Bartering with yourself and putting a time delay in can be very effective.

• Get professional help – your chances of quitting permanently are greatly improved if you have the back-up of a smoking-cessation clinic. If your doctor's surgery doesn't run one, they can advise you of local services.

📣 **DR DAWN'S HEALTH CHECK**
What happens to your body when you give up cigarettes?

Just 20 minutes after your last cigarette, your body starts to feel the benefits. Your circulation, especially to your hands and feet, improves, and your blood pressure starts to fall, and this process continues. After only:

• Eight hours – oxygen levels in the blood start to return to normal, and even at this early stage your heart attack risk is already falling.

• Twenty-four hours – the lungs start to clear out debris. One of the most common symptoms immediately after giving up is a cough. This is because smoking paralyses the tiny hairs (cilia) that line your airways and move constantly to rid your air passages of all the unwanted particles and debris. When you give up smoking, your cilia will have a big backlog to deal with.

• Two days – your sense of smell and taste improve.

• Three days – breathing is easier and your energy levels start to improve.

• Two weeks – walking and exercise get easier.

• Three months – lung efficiency can improve by as much as ten per cent.

• Five years – your risk of a heart attack has fallen by 50 per cent.

• Ten years – your risk of lung cancer has fallen by 50 per cent and the risk of a heart attack is the same as someone who has never smoked.

Worried about putting on weight?

Lots of people do. Nicotine is a mild appetite suppressant and when people give up smoking, they sometimes find their appetite increases and their taste buds recover. The best way to combat this is to focus on the health benefits of not smoking – a few extra pounds pale into insignificance compared to a lifetime of cigarette damage. And why not channel your new-found energy into an exercise programme – pick something you enjoy, and giving up smoking could actually see you lose weight!

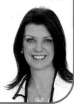

FIND OUT MORE
www.ash.org.uk
www.givingupsmoking.co.uk

CHRONIC OBSTRUCTIVE PULMONARY DISEASE

COPD for short, this is an umbrella term for a group of serious lung diseases that includes emphysema and chronic bronchitis. Chronic means long term. These conditions are almost exclusively linked to smoking, active or passive, and are, sadly, incurable. There are around three million people in the UK with COPD and around 25,000 people die of it in the UK each year.

WHAT ARE THE SYMPTOMS?

Many people with COPD find going about normal daily activities impossible because they are so short of breath – their lungs are simply too damaged to be able to provide the oxygen they need to get about.

Giving up smoking does slow down the progression of the disease, but anyone with COPD who develops a sudden deterioration in their breathing should see a doctor – flare-ups or exacerbations can lead to lengthy hospital stays.

DR DAWN'S HEALTH CHECK
If you have COPD, here are some tips to keeping well:

- Give up smoking and stay out of smoky environments.
- Don't use aerosols – most contain chemicals that can irritate your lungs.
- Have regular check-ups with the medical team looking after you.
- Never miss out your medication.
- Try to manage your stress, or better still avoid it.
- Stay as active as you can.
- Eat a healthy diet.
- Rest when you need to.
- Learn to recognize the telltale signs that your symptoms are worsening and act on them quickly.
- Have your flu vaccine every year.
- Join an easy-breathing support group – the British Lung Foundation (see website right) will be able to tell you about local services.

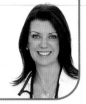

COPD is mainly a disease of smokers or those exposed to high levels of passive smoking and is thankfully rare (although not unheard of) under the age of 40. Typical symptoms include:

- A "smoker's cough" in the morning.
- Persistent coughing, often with mucus production.
- Shortness of breath on progressively less exertion.
- Recurrent chest infections, particularly in the winter.
- Wheezing or a tight chest.

A smoker with these symptoms is highly likely to have a degree of COPD, but your doctor will be able to confirm the diagnosis with a special breathing test called spirometry. You will be asked to breathe out slowly into a tube connected to a device that measures the capacity of your lungs.

WHAT CAN I DO?

Unfortunately the damage caused by COPD is irreversible, but there are a few things that may help if you do suffer from the disease:

- Stop smoking. Cutting down on the amount that you smoke isn't enough to prevent the disease from progressing, you will need to stop completely.
- Don't put any unnecessary strain on your lungs. Stay away from smoky, dusty, damp, or cold environments.
- Gentle exercise may help you to stay active, but it will not improve your lung function.

IS THERE ANY OTHER TREATMENT?

Your doctor may be able to prescribe a special inhaler to help open up the airways, and it may be necessary to use oxygen or nebulizers at home on a daily basis. However, these treatments are aimed at reducing the symptoms, and maximizing the lung function you have. They will not cure the condition.

FIND OUT MORE
www.blf-uk.org

LUNG CANCER

This illness accounts for more deaths than any other cancer in the Western world and smoking is believed to be the cause in nine out of ten cases. About 40,000 new lung cancers are diagnosed each year in the UK. Sadly, most patients put the classic symptoms of persistent cough and worsening shortness of breath down to the normal passage of smoking and don't go to their doctor until it is too late.

WHO IS AT RISK?
You could be at risk of lung cancer if you:
- Smoke, or are regularly exposed to passive smoking.
- Have worked with asbestos.
- Have been exposed to radon gas.
- Have a close relative who has had the condition.
- Have a diet lacking in fruit and vegetables. These are full of antioxidants thought to help prevent cancer, and consuming plenty of antioxidants is particularly important if you smoke.

SMOKING AND LUNG CANCER
There is no doubt that smoking is the single greatest risk factor in the development of lung cancer, but we all know people who have smoked like chimneys all their lives and escaped. The link is complicated but it seems that how long you have smoked is the key issue – if you smoke 20 cigarettes a day for 40 years your risk of developing lung cancer is eight times that of someone smoking 40 cigarettes for 20 years.

It's also a sad fact that, of the 40,000 new cases of lung cancer diagnosed this year, one in eight will not have smoked a single cigarette.

DIFFERENT TYPES OF LUNG CANCER
There are four main types of lung cancer:
- Squamous cell carcinoma.
- Small cell carcinoma.
- Adenocarcinoma.
- Large cell carcinoma.

Each type of cancer will develop in a slightly different way, so treatment will differ accordingly.

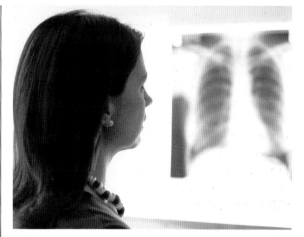
▲ A chest X-ray can be used to check for anything that looks unusual on the lung.

HOW IS IT DIAGNOSED?
A chest X-ray will normally be used to check for anything that looks unusual, or your doctor may ask you to provide a sputum sample to be examined for cancer cells. There are further lung tests that can be done in hospital if necessary.

CAN IT BE CURED?
Treatment for lung cancer will depend on the stage at which the cancer has been detected and whether the cancer has spread to other parts of the body. If lung cancer is diagnosed early, there is a much better chance of curing the condition, but as things stand, the chances of being alive five years after diagnosis are only one in 20. Remember, if you smoke it is never too late to give up (see p.70).

> **! SEEK MEDICAL ADVICE NOW**
>
> We all get coughs from time to time and most clear up without the need for any treatment, some need antibiotics, but some really shouldn't be ignored. You must see your doctor if:
> - A cough persists for several weeks.
> - You cough up blood.
> - You are short of breath.
> - You lose weight unintentionally.
> - You have a hoarse voice.

• The liver produces nearly all the proteins involved in clotting blood – without it you would bleed to death • It stores about 80g (2⅕oz) sugar in the form of glycogen for the body to use in times of starvation • Only about 20 per cent of your cholesterol comes from your diet, the other 80 per cent is made by the liver • The liver is the only organ in the body that can regenerate – from as little as 25 per cent a new liver can form • The liver is the second largest organ in the human body (the largest being the skin), and the second largest gland.

6

Liver

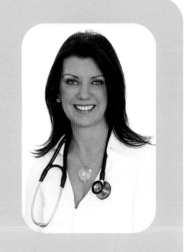

Introduction The liver is the largest internal organ in the body, weighing up to 1.5kg (3⅓lbs). It sits under your diaphragm on the right-hand side. Its lower border runs along the bottom rib but you may be surprised to learn that its upper border is approximately at the level of your nipples.

The liver is a giant filter – it breaks down poisons, such as alcohol, metabolizes most of the medicines we take, makes the proteins that help with blood clotting, and produces a substance from cholesterol called bile, which is used in the digestion of food. The bile is stored ready for use in a small organ that sits underneath the liver called the gallbladder.

Our liver is a highly sophisticated chemical processing plant. Scientists estimate that the liver performs in excess of 500 different functions, many of which are essential to life. Most of us accept that our lives depend on our lungs and hearts working properly, but our liver is so important that if it stopped working, we would die within 24 hours.

ALCOHOL AND YOUR LIVER

The liver can process (metabolize) on average one unit of alcohol an hour, but this varies greatly among different people and some regular heavy drinkers can metabolize alcohol much more quickly. However, even small amounts of alcohol can impair judgement and coordination, and large amounts may cause unconsciousness; very large amounts can even be fatal. Long-term excessive drinking may permanently damage the liver and other body systems.

HOW IS ALCOHOL CONSUMPTION MEASURED?

Alcohol is measured in units. One unit of alcohol equals 125ml (4fl oz) glass of eight per cent wine, 250ml (9fl oz) of four per cent beer, or a 25ml (1fl oz) measure of spirits. You should be aware that any home-poured drink will almost certainly be larger than these standard measures. Many pubs and bars not only now use 250ml (9fl oz) glasses as standard for wine, wine is generally much stronger than the eight per cent mentioned above!

A good way to assess how many units you consume is to look at the percentage of alcohol in the drink. This figure is the number of units in 1 litre (1¾ pints) of that drink. So if, for example, you are drinking a 12 per cent wine, then a standard 750ml (26fl oz) bottle will contain nine units of alcohol, making one large glass (250ml/9fl oz) equal to three units of alcohol.

ARE THERE SAFE ALCOHOL LIMITS?

It is recommended that women should drink no more than 14 units of alcohol a week, and men no more than 21 units. The units should be spread over the week, and ideally you should have at least two dry days a week.

Alcohol in the blood is measured as milligrams per 100ml (3½fl oz) of blood. It is difficult to equate this to units, but as a rough guide, people start to become garrulous, uninhibited, and aggressive once alcohol levels are over 100mg alcohol per 100ml of blood. Staggering and slurred speech occur after around 200mg per 100ml and levels of 400mg per 100ml can be fatal.

WHAT IS BINGE DRINKING?

It's a lot less than you think. Experts differ in their definitions, but some believe a binge to be six units in one sitting for women and eight for men. This means that a woman drinking two large glasses of 12 per cent wine in one evening is bingeing. And after an episode of drunkenness, you should give your liver 48 hours without alcohol to recover.

WHY DO SOME PEOPLE SEEM TO GET DRUNK MORE QUICKLY THAN OTHERS?

Many factors influence how quickly a person gets drunk. Drinking on an empty stomach causes the alcohol to be absorbed into the blood more quickly, and the higher the percentage of alcohol the quicker it is absorbed, so drinking wine on an empty stomach is likely to affect you more quickly than drinking beer with a curry. And warm drinks are absorbed more quickly than cold ones.

ONE UNIT OF ALCOHOL

Half a pint of beer
250ml/9fl oz
alcohol: 4%

1 small glass of wine
125ml/4fl oz
alcohol: 8%

1 single measure of spirits
25ml/1fl oz
alcohol: 40%

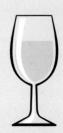

1 small glass of sherry
50ml/2fl oz
alcohol: 20%

Women tend to be more susceptible to alcohol than men, partly because they have a smaller volume of blood, and partly because they have lower levels of the enzyme that breaks alcohol down.

DRINKING TOO MUCH

Consistently drinking above the recommended limits puts you at risk of liver disease. The initial damage involves a fatty infiltration of the liver. This won't necessarily give you any symptoms so don't expect any warning signs, but the good news is that the changes are completely reversible if you stop drinking at that stage. However, if you continue to drink, you run the risk of inflammatory change to your liver, which can progress to irreversible cirrhosis of the liver and an increased risk of liver cancer.

ALCOHOL AND PREGNANCY

Drinking regularly when you are pregnant puts your unborn baby at risk of being born too small or too early. However, the jury is still out on what levels are safe – one or two units once or twice a week is unlikely to do any harm, but if you can live without drinking you are probably better off to abstain from alcohol altogether.

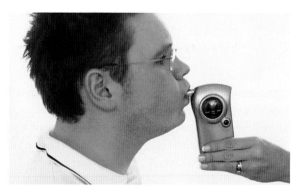

▲ *A breathalyser can give a reliable measure of the amount of alcohol in your bloodstream.*

AVOIDING A HANGOVER

- Eat before you go out.
- Stick to pale drinks.
- Limit yourself to one unit an hour.
- Alternate any alcoholic drinks with water or soft drinks.
- Don't stay up too late.
- Drink fruit juice high in vitamin C before you go to bed.

? DID YOU KNOW
Drinking and driving

Undoubtedly the best thing is not to drink at all if you are going to be driving. Alcohol slows down your reactions, affects your judgement, and makes you more likely to take risks. The actual legal limit for driving varies from country to country, but in the UK it is 80mg alcohol per 100ml (3½fl oz) blood.

How much can I drink and still be under the limit for driving?

Unfortunately, there is no hard and fast rule on this one. So many factors influence how quickly your body absorbs (and clears) alcohol. This varies not only from person to person, but also from day to day for any individual. A 51kg (8 stone) woman could be over the limit after one large glass of wine if she is drinking on an empty stomach. The best answer is to avoid alcohol altogether or to use a hand-held breathalyser.

DR DAWN'S HEALTH CHECK
What defines a drink problem?

How much you drink, why you drink, and whether or not you depend on alcohol are important factors when identifying a drinking problem. Start by asking yourself the following questions:

- Have you ever felt you should cut down your drinking?
- Have you ever been annoyed about others criticizing your drinking?
- Have you ever felt guilty or ashamed about your drinking?
- Have you ever had an alcoholic drink as an eye-opener to face the day?

If you answered yes to any two or more, the chances are you may have a problem.

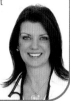

FIND OUT MORE
www.alcoholconcern.org.uk
www.downyourdrink.org.uk

MYTH BUSTERS
Let's take a look at some of the myths that we hear about alcohol.

DRINKING VODKA AND CHAMPAGNE WON'T GIVE YOU A HANGOVER

TRUE

Well, within reason! As a rough guide, paler drinks contain fewer congeners (the chemicals in alcoholic drinks partly responsible for the symptoms of a hangover). They are not the whole story, but, unit for unit, you are likely to feel better the morning after if you stick to pale alcoholic drinks.

MIXING YOUR DRINKS GIVES YOU A WORSE HANGOVER

FALSE

It's not the mixture itself that causes the problem. The more types of alcoholic drinks you have in an evening, the more likely you are to be drinking darker drinks containing the congeners that make you more prone to hangovers.

DRINKING THROUGH A STRAW WILL GET YOU DRUNK MORE QUICKLY

FALSE

The only alcoholic drinks you generally drink through straws are cocktails. They may get you drunk quickly but it has nothing to do with the straw and everything to do with the high alcohol content of cocktails.

DRINKING COFFEE AT THE END OF THE EVENING WILL SOBER YOU UP

FALSE

Caffeine has no effect on blood-alcohol levels; it's a stimulant so it can make you feel less drowsy, but don't rely on it if you are thinking of driving.

YOU CANNOT DRINK ALCOHOL WHILE TAKING ANTIBIOTICS

FALSE

Alcohol within the recommended limits won't interfere with most antibiotics. However, there is one antibiotic, metronidazole, that is chemically similar to a drug (called disulfiram) used to help people who are dependent on alcohol stay off the drink. People who drink alcohol when taking metronidazole run the risk of very unpleasant effects, including a blinding headache and possibly nausea and vomiting.

HAIR OF THE DOG WILL CURE A HANGOVER

TRUE

But it's not to be recommended! Some of the products of alcohol that cause the symptoms of a hangover can be knocked off their receptors if you drink more alcohol, but you are only delaying the inevitable. If you have a hangover, you almost certainly drank enough for it to be classified as a binge the night before and you should give your liver a rest.

ALCOHOL HELPS YOU TO SLEEP BETTER

FALSE

Alcohol is a sedative. It may help you get off to sleep, but then it interferes with your normal sleep patterns, meaning you get less deep "battery-recharging" sleep – this is one reason why you feel so dreadful the following day.

GALLSTONES

These are small "stones" that form in the gallbladder. Around one in five UK adults has gallstones, but only five per cent cause symptoms, which classically include pain in the upper right side of your abdomen. The pain is typically worse after eating fatty foods and is often associated with sickness.

WHO IS AT RISK?

When I was at medical school we were taught that gallstones were a disease of the "fair, fat, and forty". Not much has changed, although we are more politically correct! Gallstones are more common in women than men, and obesity is still one of the biggest risk factors.

WHAT CAN BE DONE

You may be able to prevent gallstones from developing in the first place by cutting down on fatty foods and maintaining a healthy weight. If you do get gallstones that cause symptoms, there are drugs that can dissolve the stones but success rates are less than 50 per cent. Most people opt for an operation to remove the gallbladder. This can be done by keyhole (laparoscopic) surgery and, provided there are no complications, most patients make a full recovery within two weeks.

▾ *An ultrasound scan showing a large gallstone (red area) in the gallbladder.*

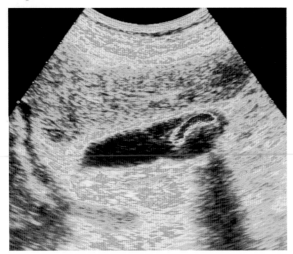

CIRRHOSIS

Cirrhosis occurs when the normal liver tissue is replaced by scar tissue, which prevents the normal flow of blood through the organ and prevents it from functioning properly. The most common causes of cirrhosis in the UK are heavy alcohol consumption and hepatitis C infection. The liver has amazing powers of regeneration but when it is so damaged that cirrhosis develops, it cannot recover.

WHAT ARE THE SYMPTOMS?

In the early stages of cirrhosis you may continue to feel relatively well, but as the condition progresses symptoms develop, including:
- Jaundice (yellow tinge to the skin and whites of the eyes).
- Lethargy and confusion.
- Nausea, loss of appetite, and weight loss.
- Swollen ankles due to fluid retention.
- Itching.

HOW IS CIRRHOSIS DIAGNOSED?

If your doctor suspects cirrhosis, they will probably arrange blood tests in the first instance. If these confirm liver damage, an ultrasound or CT scan will show the damage, and you may also have a biopsy, in which cells are removed from the liver under local anaesthetic and examined for clues about the cause of the damage.

CAN CIRRHOSIS BE TREATED?

Cirrhosis is serious, irreversible, and, in half of those diagnosed with cirrhosis today, fatal within five years. The only cure is to have a liver transplant, but there are several things that you can do to help yourself:
- Stop drinking alcohol – continuing to drink at this stage is signing your own death warrant. Cut it out completely.
- Ask your doctor or pharmacist about any medicines that you are taking, including those bought over the counter. If you have serious liver damage, your body may no longer be able to cope with them. Your doctor will be able to advise on whether they should be stopped altogether or whether the dose simply needs to be reduced.
- A low-salt diet will help reduce fluid retention.

HEPATITIS

This means inflammation of the liver. There are three main types of infective hepatitis that I will look at – hepatitis A, B, and C.

HEPATITIS A

This is the mildest form of hepatitis. It is usually caught from contaminated food or drink. The incubation period is anything from two to six weeks. Symptoms start with a flu-like illness and fatigue, followed several days later by dark urine, jaundice (yellow hue to the skin and whites of the eyes), and pale faeces. Most people recover without needing treatment, but adults with the disease should avoid alcohol and the oral contraceptive pill until blood tests show the liver has returned to normal, which can take several months. You can be vaccinated against

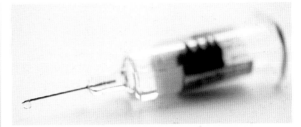
▲ Hepatitis B and C can be caught from infected needles.

hepatitis A – anyone travelling to high-risk areas should ask their doctor about it. While abroad, wash fruit and salad in bottled or boiled water, not tap water.

HEPATITIS B

This is a much more serious infection transmitted by blood contact or sexual intercourse. The virus can also survive on surfaces outside the body for up to a week. The incubation period for hepatitis B is three to six months, which means that you can pass on the infection before you know you have it. Unlike hepatitis A, the B virus can cause chronic infection, with a risk of developing cirrhosis. Again, there is a vaccine for hepatitis B if you are in one of the at-risk groups.

DOS AND DON'TS IF YOU HAVE HEPATITIS B
- Do use condoms for oral or penetrative sex.
- Don't share razor blades, toothbrushes, or anything that may be contaminated with body fluids.
- Don't share needles if you are injecting drugs.

HEPATITIS C

Like hepatitis B, hepatitis C is carried in the blood. Most people with hepatitis C do not have any symptoms, and about one in four infected people clears the virus from their body without long-term problems. However, left untreated, there is a one in five chance of developing cirrhosis, so if you are in an at-risk group, you should talk to your doctor about having a blood test to check it out.

> **? DID YOU KNOW**
> **Who is at risk?**
>
> The following groups are at risk of hepatitis B:
> - Injecting drug users who share needles.
> - Health-care professionals.
> - People who travel frequently to areas such as Southeast Asia and Africa.
> - Sexual and household contacts of hepatitis B carriers.
> - Men who have sex with men.
> - People who frequently change their sexual partners.
>
> If you fall into any of these groups you should consider vaccination, involving a course of three injections. It is important to have a blood test after the final injection as one in ten people will need a booster.
>
> The following groups are at risk of hepatitis C:
> - Injecting drug users who share needles.
> - People who received a blood transfusion before 1991 (since then all blood has been screened for hepatitis C).
> - Babies born to hepatitis C-positive mothers.
> - People who have a tattoo or piercing done with infected equipment.
> - People who share razors or toothbrushes.
> - People who have medical or dental treatment in parts of the world where the virus is common and sterilization techniques may not be adequate.

> **FIND OUT MORE**
> **www.britishlivertrust.org.uk**
> **www.hep-ccentre.com**

• The average adult digestive system is 8 to 9m (26 to 30ft) long • The surface of the intestine has millions of tiny folds – if it didn't contain these folds, your intestine would need to be 3.2km (2 miles) long to work as effectively • Food takes up to three days to travel from your mouth to your anus • In an average lifetime, a gut will handle around 65 tonnes of food and drink – that is approximately the weight of 8 double-decker buses • Your gut contains around 1.8kg (4lbs) of living bacteria from about 400 different species of friendly bacteria called "gut flora".

7

Digestive system

Introduction Our digestive system is a complex piece of machinery, combining the intricate actions of muscles, nerves, hormones, and secretions to keep everything working properly.

Your gastrointestinal system is one long muscular tube. When food enters the mouth and is swallowed it enters the oesophagus, where it sets up a wave of contractions, propelling it through the system. When food reaches the stomach, hydrochloric acid and digestive enzymes start to break it down, and smaller molecules, such as alcohol and glucose, are absorbed into the bloodstream. The rest of the food is then passed to the small intestine, which has three parts – the duodenum, the jejunum and the ileum. The small intestine is where most of the digestive processes occur and where most of the nutrients are absorbed.

From here, what is left is passed on to the large intestine which also has three parts – the caecum, the colon and the rectum. It is in the large intestine that water is reabsorbed into the body, leaving what we recognize as faeces to pass into the rectum.

INDIGESTION

Sometimes called heartburn, indigestion is so common that at any one time about one in four of people are suffering from it, and nearly everyone will experience it at some time in their lives. Indigestion is caused by an upset in the normal acidic conditions of the intestine: too much acid, acid in the wrong place, or inadequate protection from acid in the stomach lining.

WHAT CAUSES IT?

There are many possible causes of indigestion; the more common ones include:

- Stress.
- Smoking.
- Drinking alcohol, especially drinking too much.
- Caffeine consumption – coffee, tea, and cola drinks.
- Overeating, especially eating too much rich food.
- Weight gain.
- Pregnancy.
- Medications, such as anti-inflammatories and steroids.
- Infection with *Helicobacter pylori* bacteria.

WHAT YOU CAN DO

So what can you do if you are one of the millions of adults who suffer from indigestion, and when should you get medical advice? The first step for anyone who often gets indigestion is to look at their lifestyle. If you smoke, then stop; cut down on your alcohol and caffeine intake; and lose weight if your body mass index (BMI) is over 25 (see p.94). If you are also under a lot of stress, you should look at ways of managing it, which is perhaps the most difficult aspect of your lifestyle to tackle. Try keeping a diary of the things that stress you; some you won't be able to do anything about, but writing it down will help you to see more clearly the things you can change.

Indigestion caused by *Helicobacter pylori* – a common bacteria – can often be cured with a short course of antibiotics and medicines called proton-pump inhibitors, or PPIs (see below).

The vast majority of people manage their symptoms by simple adjustments to their lifestyle and using over-the-counter remedies, but there are some symptoms you shouldn't ignore (see box below).

HOW DO THE DRUG TREATMENTS WORK?

There are four main classes of drugs available for the treatment of indigestion, and the first two are available from your chemist. They include:

- Antacids – these neutralize the acid. They work quickly but stop working when your stomach empties.
- Alginates – these form a raft over the contents of your stomach, to keep the acid contained. They work quickly but as soon as you eat again your stomach produces more acid on top and the effect is lost.
- H2 receptor antagonists – these reduce the amount of acid produced. They take longer to act but the effect can last for up to 12 hours.
- Proton-pump inhibitors (PPIs) – these drugs switch off acid production in your stomach. They are long-lasting and extremely effective.

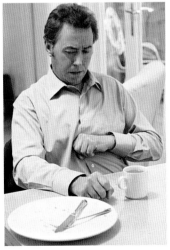

◄ *Eating too much rich, spicy, or fatty food is a common cause of indigestion.*

> **! SEEK MEDICAL ADVICE NOW**
> **If you have any of the following:**
>
> - You cannot control your symptoms with lifestyle changes and over-the-counter remedies.
> - You have unintentional weight loss.
> - Food feels as if it's getting stuck in your gullet.
> - You vomit blood.
> - Your stools have turned black (this can be a sign that they contain blood from the stomach).
> - You develop new symptoms and are over 55.

PEPTIC ULCERS

An ulcer forms where there is damage to the lining of the stomach or first part of the intestine (duodenum). When I was working as a junior hospital doctor, we used to admit at least one person every day with bleeding from a stomach or duodenal ulcer. However, this is a medical emergency that I haven't seen in years.

WHY ARE THEY NOW RARE?

I put it down to a combination of a better understanding of what causes ulcers and some excellent new drugs. Doctors are acutely aware of the link between anti-inflammatory drugs (a group of drugs that includes aspirin and ibuprofen) and stomach irritation, so we stop them at the first sign of indigestion, before more damage can be done. This, and the introduction of the proton-pump inhibitor drugs, which switch off acid production in the stomach, has meant that ulcers are now rare.

EARLY WARNING SIGNS

Although ulcers are rare today, it is important to be aware of early warning signs so that you can see your doctor for treatment before an ulcer develops.

The main early warning sign is persistent or repeated bouts of indigestion, particularly if there is no obvious cause for them, such as overeating or drinking too much. other signs to look out for include nausea and/or vomiting, loss of appetite, and unintentional weight loss.

FLATULENCE

A burp is the emission of gas from the mouth and it is rarely significant medically but can be embarrassing. The gas emitted is usually air but it often brings with it the smell of partly digested food in the stomach.

WHAT YOU CAN DO

Here are a couple of things you can do to reduce burps:
- Don't bolt your food.
- Avoid carbonated drinks. The fizz has to go somewhere.

THE OTHER END

The gas emitted when we break wind is different – it's not made up of the air we swallow but is a collection of gas bubbles produced in the colon by the action of bacteria on the food. We produce 200ml–2 litres (7–70 fl oz) of gas in this way each day, and the quantity increases dramatically with certain foods, especially cabbage, onions, and pulses. If you suppress the urge to break wind, the gas is reabsorbed harmlessly by your gut.

▾ Cabbage and some other vegetables produce large amounts of intestinal gas while they are being digested.

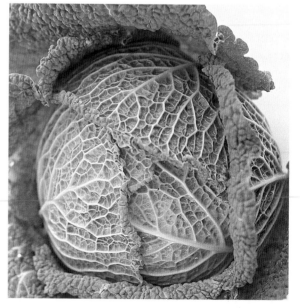

CONSTIPATION

This simply means opening your bowels less often than usual and/or having to strain to pass faeces. The word "usual" is important here, because what is normal can vary hugely from person to person; it can be anything from two to three times a day, to two to three times a week. For instance, if you normally open your bowels twice a day, then only opening them twice a week could mean that you are constipated.

WHAT CAUSES IT?

Your intestine is basically a long muscular tube along which food is propelled by muscular contraction – a bit like squeezing toothpaste. Water and nutrients are extracted from the food along the way, and its progress is influenced by many factors. Changes to anything that influences your bowel action may lead to constipation, including:

• Diet – not having enough fibre in your diet or not drinking enough fluids.

• Poor bowel habit – mainly ignoring the urge to open your bowels.

• Age – older people are more prone to constipation.

• Exercise – the less active we are, the less active our bowels are too.

• Medication – many drugs, including some painkillers, antidepressants, and diuretics (water pills), may cause constipation. If you have noticed a problem since starting a new medication, talk to your doctor – there may be an alternative. But never stop taking any prescribed medication without consulting your doctor.

• Hormonal changes – especially in pregnancy.

• Travel – the combination of a change in diet and schedule when on holiday can make some people constipated, although the reverse is more common.

• Medical problems – particularly hypothyroidism (an underactive thyroid gland).

WHAT YOU CAN DO

If changes to your diet and lifestyle that address the possible causes don't seem to work, medication may help. Many constipation medications are available without

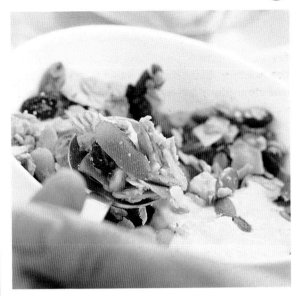

▲ *Muesli and other high-fibre foods can help prevent constipation.*

prescription from your chemist, but the differences between them can be confusing; ask your pharmacist if in doubt. Broadly, such medications can be divided into four categories:

• Bulk-forming laxatives – these are good for people who cannot get enough fibre in their diet and have an ongoing problem with constipation. These laxatives may take several days to work and can cause bloating and wind.

• Faecal softeners – these, as the name suggests, soften your faeces, making them easier to pass.

• Osmotic laxatives – these work by drawing fluid from your body and retaining it in your bowel.

• Stimulant laxatives – these work by increasing bowel contractions; they start to take effect within a few hours.

! SEEK MEDICAL ADVICE NOW
If you have tried the simple lifestyle changes and/or over-the-counter or home remedies and:

• Constipation persists for several weeks.

• You pass blood in your faeces.

• You lose weight unintentionally.

• You have severe abdominal pain.

• You also have diarrhoea.

PILES (HAEMORRHOIDS)

These are similar to varicose veins but are in the anus, the last part of the intestine. Piles are very common: half of us will have them at some time in our lives. They are often caused by straining to open your bowels, which itself may be due to constipation. In pregnant women, the pressure exerted by a growing fetus is a common cause.

WHAT ARE THE SYMPTOMS?

Often there are no symptoms at all, but you may notice a lump around your anus, itching, or fresh red bleeding from your anus. It may also be uncomfortable when you open your bowels. Occasionally, a thrombus (blood clot) can form in a pile. Unlike most other clots, this isn't dangerous but it can be painful.

SHOULD YOU GET MEDICAL ADVICE?

Yes, you should talk to your doctor. A small pile that isn't causing any problems might not need any treatment. If your doctor does recommend treatment, it usually starts with creams and suppositories and this might be all that is needed. However, if such treatment doesn't work, more aggressive treatment may be necessary. This may involve one of the following:
• Injecting a pile with a chemical to make it shrink.
• Putting a tiny elastic band around the base of a pile so that it eventually drops off.

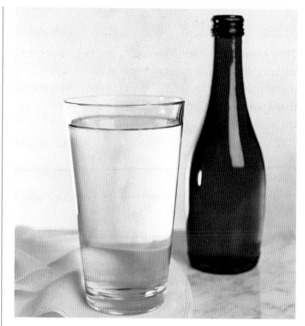

▲ *Drinking plenty of water - at least eight glasses a day - can help reduce the likelihood of developing piles.*

• Freezing it off (cryotherapy).
In extreme cases, your doctor may recommend that you have an operation under general anaesthetic to have the piles removed (haemorrhoidectomy).

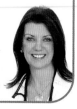

DR DAWN'S HEALTH CHECK
How to reduce your risk of developing piles:
• Never strain to open your bowels.
• Go to the toilet when you need to – don't hold it in.
• Have plenty of fibre in your diet.
• Drink at least eight glasses of fluids each day.
• Take regular exercise.
Some people ask me if sitting on cold seats can give you piles. The answer is that sitting down for long periods can make you more prone to piles, but the temperature of what you sit on is irrelevant.

 DID YOU KNOW
Anal itching
Itching around the anus is rarely serious but may be embarrassing. Common causes include poor personal hygiene, piles (haemorrhoids), worms, or allergy to a product such as soap. It may also occur with some skin diseases, such as eczema or psoriasis. If careful washing with hypoallergenic soap or use of an over-the-counter steroid cream doesn't stop the itching within a few days, you should see your doctor.

FIND OUT MORE
www.digestivedisorders.co.uk

DIARRHOEA

This condition is defined as passing loose or watery faeces and/or more frequent bowel movements than usual. As with constipation, the frequency of bowel movements depends on what is normal for you.

WHAT YOU CAN DO

Most diarrhoeal illnesses are short-lived and can be treated by increasing your fluid intake to avoid becoming dehydrated and taking over-the-counter medicines to stop the diarrhoea. A word of warning here though – try to avoid taking antidiarrhoeal medicines during the first 24 hours of the illness. This is because diarrhoea is often caused by a bug and preventing the bugs from coming out of your system may make you feel more unwell in the longer term. Most of the infected faeces will have left your intestine within about 24 hours, although many people continue to pass loose faeces for some time afterwards. This can be because, along with all the bad bugs, you have lost much of your natural gut flora (the beneficial bacteria that normally live in your intestines). Taking an antidiarrhoeal medicine at this second stage in the illness can help these good bacteria to multiply and repopulate your intestines.

PROBIOTICS CAN HELP RECOVERY

We know that our natural gut flora play a vital role in the digestion of foods that we cannot break down on our own, and in the absorption of vitamins and minerals in food. Gut flora also help break down toxins and keep bad bacteria like those responsible for food poisoning at bay. A probiotic is a mixture of live bacteria (usually from the *Lactobacillus* or *Bifidobacterium* groups) that can be taken as yoghurt drinks, pills, or even as a cereal. Experts differ in their advice regarding probiotics, but my view is that it stands to reason that if you are rapidly losing your own good bacteria through diarrhoea, then replacing them with a probiotic until your body has had a chance to recover makes a lot of sense.

HOW DO I KNOW IF I AM DEHYDRATED?

If diarrhoea persists, is severe, or is accompanied by fever, there is a danger of losing too much fluid and

essential body salts – this is dehydration. Doctors have various ways of assessing dehydration but, as a rough guide, keep an eye on the colour of your urine – it should be pale or straw-coloured. If it becomes very dark, you are probably becoming dehydrated and should increase your fluid intake (see Dealing with diarrhoea, below). If this doesn't work, talk to your doctor.

DR DAWN'S HEALTH CHECK
Dealing with diarrhoea

If you have diarrhoea make sure that:

- You increase your fluid intake to 3–4 litres (5–7 pints) per day. I often advise patients to drink flat cola or lemonade as it will give you some sugar, or you can buy sachets of rehydration salts from your chemist.
- You are extra vigilant about washing your hands, particularly before eating and after every visit to the toilet.
- Once you feel better, you start taking a probiotic daily to recolonize your gut with good bacteria.
- Eat as soon as your appetite returns but keep your diet bland to start with.
- Take paracetamol if you have a fever – a temperature rise of just one degree results in an extra 500ml (18 fl oz) of sweat and makes you more prone to dehydration.

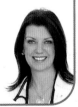

! SEEK MEDICAL ADVICE NOW
If along with your diarrhoea:

- You have a high fever and feel unwell.
- You have blood or pus in the diarrhoea.
- You have recently returned from foreign travel.
- Your symptoms have persisted for more than a week.
- You are becoming dehydrated, even after you have increased you fluid intake as mentioned above.

IRRITABLE BOWEL SYNDROME

Often called IBS, this condition affects about one in five people in the UK and is more common in women than men. The symptoms tend to come on intermittently but may persist for many years.

WHAT ARE THE SYMPTOMS?

The most common symptoms of IBS are painful abdominal spasms, bloating, and increased wind. Some people also have diarrhoea, which may alternate with periods of constipation, and sometimes nausea and vomiting. Typically, the symptoms recur intermittently and the condition may last for years. However, the symptoms and pattern of recurrence of attacks tend to vary widely, both among different people and even in the same person at different times.

The symptoms are thought to be caused either by stronger than normal muscle contractions of the colon or by a heightened awareness of normal contractions. Either way, a diagnosis of IBS is made only after excluding other possible causes of the symptoms. There is no single test or scan that can confirm the condition.

WHAT YOU CAN DO

There isn't a cure for IBS but a few lifestyle changes can make a significant impact on symptoms. Diet and stress play a major role in IBS, and I often find it useful to get patients to keep a food diary for a few weeks. Writing down everything you eat and when your symptoms occur can be enlightening. If your food diary suggests a link with a particular food group (say, dairy products or wheat, which are common IBS triggers), it is worth excluding that group from your diet for a few weeks. I am not generally keen on exclusion diets unless they are absolutely necessary, and because we know that stress and routine can also be factors, it may be worth reintroducing the excluded foods after a time to see how you react. If your symptoms disappeared and then recur, and you want to exclude a food group long term, speak to a dietitian for advice on how to replace the nutrients that it provided.

Stress is less easy to pinpoint, but again keeping a diary can be useful – many IBS sufferers are juggling home and work lives and sometimes it's only when you write everything down that you can spot areas of stress. Of course, some stresses can't be avoided but a diary may help identify the ones you can do something about.

WHAT ELSE CAN I DO?

• Drink more water. Dehydration can make the symptoms of IBS worse.

• Consider including a daily probiotic in your diet. Available as tablets, cereals, or drinks – many IBS sufferers find them helpful.

• Talk to your doctor about medication to ease the pain of the bowel spasms.

▼ *Painful abdominal spasms are a common symptom of IBS.*

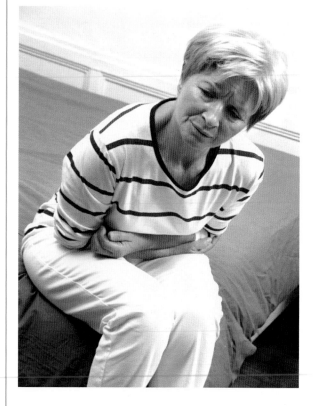

FIND OUT MORE
www.ibsgroup.org

HERNIAS

A hernia (popularly known as a rupture) is simply a protrusion of part of the bowel through a weakness in the muscular wall of the abdomen.

SITES OF HERNIAS

Common sites include the groin (these are called inguinal or femoral hernias) and around the navel (called umbilical hernias). Umbilical hernias are common in pregnant or overweight women and babies may sometimes be born with them, whereas inguinal hernias are more common in men. Many hernias just appear when we strain, when lifting a heavy weight or passing a bowel movement, for example. If a hernia can be pushed back in (reduced), then you may not need treatment but it should still be checked by your doctor.

WILL YOU NEED SURGERY?

Once a hernia has developed, the only way to get rid of it permanently is with surgery. However, not everybody needs surgery and some people opt to wear a truss to help support the muscles.

The main risk is that a hernia will become strangulated (meaning it can't be pushed back). This is a painful condition that needs urgent surgery to prevent the protruding part of the bowel from dying. Interestingly, the smaller the hernia, the greater the risk of strangulation; large hernias may look more unsightly but are less likely to strangulate.

? DID YOU KNOW

Who is at risk?

Men are more prone to inguinal hernias than women because when the testicles drop into the scrotal sac, they leave a weakness in the groin that women don't have. Beyond that, anything that puts extra strain on the muscles of the abdominal wall increases the risk. Common examples include:

- Pregnancy.
- Constipation, and straining to pass faeces.
- Heavy lifting.
- Persistent coughing.

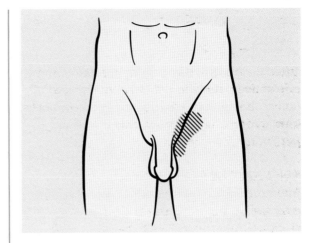

▲ *Site of an inguinal hernia.*

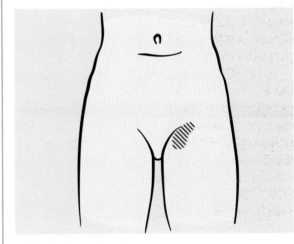

▲ *Site of a femoral hernia.*

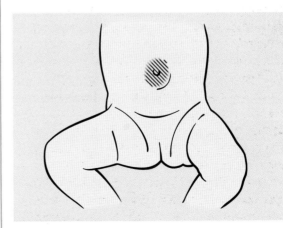

▲ *Site of an umbilical hernia.*

FOOD ALLERGY AND INTOLERANCE

More than one in three of the population claims to have a food allergy but the real figure is nearer one in fifty. It has become trendy to blame food allergy for anything from weight gain to poor complexion and loss of libido, but it's important to distinguish true allergy, which is potentially life-threatening, from intolerance, which is not.

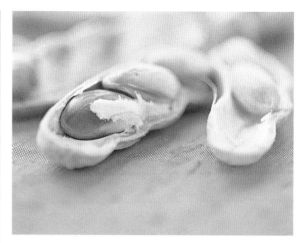

▲ Peanuts are one of the most common food allergens.

FOOD ALLERGY SYMPTOMS

A food allergy is an immune-mediated reaction to food, and its symptoms range from an itchy skin rash that looks as if you have been stung by nettles (urticaria), nausea, vomiting, and diarrhoea to life-threatening anaphylaxis, when you suffer dramatic swelling of the lips, tongue and throat, and severe wheezing within about an hour of contact with the allergen. Allergies tend to become worse with repeated exposure and it's therefore important to receive a clear diagnosis so you can avoid the allergen in future.

COMMON FOOD ALLERGENS

The foods that most commonly trigger an allergic reaction include:

- Peanuts and tree nuts.
- Cow's milk.
- Hen's eggs.
- Fish and shellfish.
- Soya.
- Wheat.
- Citrus fruits and strawberries.

Identification of a specific allergen is usually made on the basis of the patient's case history but it may be confirmed with blood tests or skin prick tests.

WHY IS PEANUT ALLERGY SO COMMON?

Peanut allergy was almost unheard of when I was at school and yet today many schools are "nut-free", and you can barely get on a plane without being asked to refrain from eating nuts because someone on board has such a severe allergy that exposure to the tiniest amount could cause a life-threatening reaction.

One theory to explain the huge increase in peanut allergy in the last 20 years is that there has been an enormous increase in the use of peanut oil and peanut derivatives in packaged foods. Some scientists believe that high exposure to peanut while in the womb may cause allergy later in life. This theory has not yet been proved but I certainly advise my pregnant and breastfeeding patients to avoid peanut products.

WHAT TO DO IF SOMEONE HAS AN ALLERGIC REACTION

The action to take depends on the severity of the reaction. If you have any antihistamine to hand, you should give it to the person immediately. If the person has a very severe, life-threatening reaction (anaphylaxis), this is a medical emergency and you should follow the instructions in the box below.

! EMERGENCY – DIAL 999

Allergic reactions can develop rapidly into anaphylaxis, when the lips and tongue swell and the person has difficulty breathing. If this occurs:

- It is a medical emergency and you will need to get medical help as quickly as possible; if necessary call an ambulance.
- If the person has an autoinjector, help him or her administer it, or give it yourself if you know how.

WHAT IS FOOD INTOLERANCE?

Food intolerance is much more common than food allergy, affecting as many as one person in five. The symptoms of intolerance are often vague and include abdominal pain and bloating, nausea, and constipation or diarrhoea. The key differences between food intolerance and allergy are the time scale and variability. People who are intolerant to a food usually develop symptoms hours or even days after exposure to it and may go through phases when they are able to tolerate it again. In contrast, allergic symptoms come on more rapidly – within about an hour of exposure to the allergen – and occur every time the allergen is encountered.

WHAT YOU CAN DO ABOUT INTOLERANCE

Keeping a food and symptom diary can help you identify foods that you might be intolerant to. If you notice a pattern, try eliminating that food from your diet for a few weeks and continue to keep a symptom diary. If your symptoms definitely improve, you could be intolerant, but always reintroduce the food for a while to see if your symptoms recur. If they do and you are considering eliminating the food long term, it is important to consult a dietitian to make sure you replace the nutrients that you would be missing. And remember, many food intolerances are transient so it is worth challenging your system again at a later date.

LACTOSE INTOLERANCE

The inability to digest lactose, the natural sugar found in milk and dairy products, is so common in certain groups of people that it's debatable whether it's a disease or not. About eight out of ten adults of African, Asian, Native American, or Jewish origin have it, but it is rare in those of northern European origin.

The condition is due to lack of an enzyme that normally digests lactose in the intestines. As a result, undigested lactose builds up, leading to abdominal pain, bloating, and diarrhoea. These symptoms usually come on a few hours after eating or drinking food products containing milk. Fortunately, lactose intolerance is rare in babies and children, because high levels of the enzyme are usually present at birth. The enzyme levels gradually drop off with age and by adolescence are usually so low that lactose cannot be digested and symptoms appear.

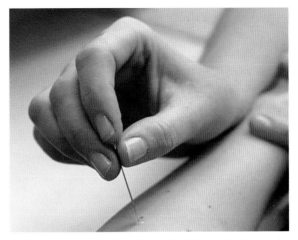

▲ A skin prick test may be used to identify specific allergens.

The symptoms of lactose intolerance can be avoided by eliminating milk and dairy products from your diet. Your doctor may also suggest that you take supplements of the missing enzyme.

FIND OUT MORE
www.allergyuk.org

? DID YOU KNOW

Why do our stomachs rumble when we are hungry?

About 12 hours after eating a meal, strong waves of muscular contraction start in the stomach and progress along the full length of the gut. They are sometimes referred to as "housekeeping movements" and can take 90 minutes to go from one end to the other before starting again. The contractions push air and fluid through the empty intestine, causing what we recognize as stomach rumblings.

Why do we feel sleepy after a big meal?

Eating carbohydrate stimulates the release of a chemical in the brain called serotonin, which makes us feel relaxed and contented.

OBESITY

The UK is the fattest nation in Europe – half the population is overweight. The heavier you are, the more likely you are to suffer from high blood pressure, raised cholesterol, heart disease, stroke, diabetes (even in children), arthritis, and even depression and infertility, not to mention some cancers, including cancer of the breast, colon, kidney, prostate, and uterus.

HOW DO I KNOW IF I AM OVERWEIGHT?

Weight is often assessed using a measure called the body mass index (BMI), which gives an indication of how much you weigh in relation to your height.

You can calculate your BMI by dividing your weight (in kilograms) by the square of your height (in metres), that is, weight (in kilograms) divided by (height in metres x height in metres) = BMI. For example, a man who weighs 75kg (11st 11lb) and is 1.8m (5ft 11in) tall has a BMI of 75 ÷ (1.8m x 1.8m = 3.24) = 23.

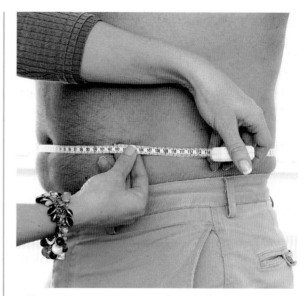

▲ Your waist measurement can give an indication of whether you have too much abdominal fat.

INTERPRETING YOUR BMI RESULT

Doctors have classified the BMI figures into five ranges:
- A BMI less than 18.5 is classed as underweight.
- A BMI between 18.5 and 24.9 is classed as a healthy weight.
- A BMI between 25 and 29.9 is classed as overweight.
- A BMI between 30 and 39.9 is classed as obese.
- A BMI of 40 or more is classed as morbidly obese.

However, these BMI figures apply to average adults under the age of 60 who are not pregnant or breastfeeding and do not have any chronic (long term) health problems (diabetes, for example). The figures are not applicable to children; nor are they applicable to people with a high proportion of body muscle, such as athletes and weight trainers.

WHERE YOU CARRY YOUR WEIGHT MATTERS

It's not just how much you weigh that's important; where you carry it is also significant. People who carry their weight mainly around their midriff (so-called "apples") are more at risk of heart disease than people who carry their weight around their hips ("pears").

In fact, the link between waist circumference and risk of coronary heart disease is so strong that some doctors are moving away from BMI as a measurement of risk to simply measuring waists.

DR DAWN'S HEALTH CHECK
Where is your weight?

Measure your waist and see below to assess your health risk, and no cheating ... I see lots of men in 90cm (36in) waist trousers that fit neatly on their hips below a 105cm (42in) beer belly of a waist. To measure your waist, stand in a relaxed posture and measure around just above your hip bone (usually around the navel); you should measure over bare skin, not over clothing, and you shouldn't hold in your stomach!

Moderate risk of heart disease or diabetes
Waist measurement:
Women between 80cm (32in) and 88cm (35in).
Men between 92cm (37in) and 100cm (40in).

Severe risk of heart disease or diabetes
Waist measurement:
Women above 88cm (35in).
Men above 100cm (40in).

THE BENEFITS OF LOSING WEIGHT

If you are obese, or even significantly overweight, the idea of achieving a size 12 or 14 (or, for men, an 82cm/32in waist) can seem so far off it's too daunting to even try, but losing just ten per cent of your body weight can have dramatic health benefits. For example, such a weight loss can result in:

- A 10mmHg drop in your blood pressure.
- A ten per cent fall in your cholesterol level.
- A 20 per cent reduction in your risk of premature death.

HOW TO LOSE WEIGHT SAFELY

The key to losing weight safely and then keeping at your lower weight is to make small changes in your diet and lifestyle that you can maintain over the long term.

So, what does this mean in practical terms? To begin with, anybody who is severely overweight should see his or her doctor, who may check that there is no underlying medical cause for your excess weight, check that there is no medical reason why you shouldn't exercise, and refer you to a dietitian for advice. If you are only slightly or moderately overweight and otherwise healthy, you should increase your activity level by taking more exercise and reduce the energy content of your diet.

▾ *Encouraging your child to be physically active can help prevent him or her from becoming overweight.*

Generally, reducing your daily energy intake to between 500 and 1,000 kcal less than the average requirement for somebody of your sex, age, and height should lead to a slow but sustainable weight loss. However, it is important that your lower-energy diet is properly balanced, with the right amount of essential nutrients. The typical Western diet contains too much fat, so you might find that the easiest way to reduce your energy intake is to cut down on fatty foods. A small amount of fat contains a lot of calories so reducing your fat intake by even a relatively small amount will reduce your energy intake significantly.

WHAT ABOUT OBESE CHILDREN?

In the UK, at least one in five children is overweight and one in ten is obese. This is a worrying statistic and it is due to a combination of too much fast food and sweet

> **? DID YOU KNOW**
> ### Weight gain can be deceptive
> A student walking 0.8km (½ mile) to college and back five days a week, burns 100 kcal per day during the walk. Over three 12-week terms, this adds up to burning 18,000 kcal a year – that's equivalent to 2.2kg (5lb) of fat. If the student leaves college at 22 weighing 70kg (11st), buys a car and doesn't compensate for this reduction in energy expenditure in any other way, by the time he is 30 he will weigh 89kg (14st).

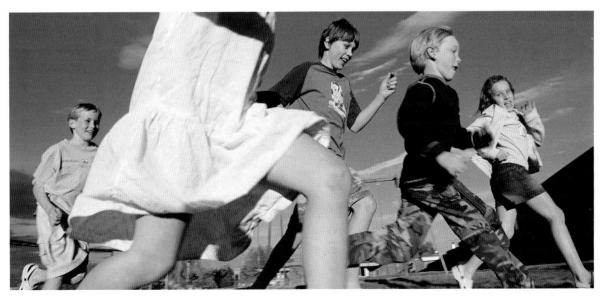

drinks in their diets, larger portion sizes, and less active lifestyles. So, what should you do if your child is on the tubby side and when should you worry?

It's normal to carry some "puppy fat" in our early years but as a general rule, I think children should be slimming down by the time they start junior school (around eight years of age) and children who are still overweight by the age of 11 really worry me – they are far more likely to remain an unhealthy weight throughout adulthood.

I'm not too keen on diets in children. Growing children need a balanced diet and, to be honest, it's impossible to get all but the most motivated of children to stick to a diet. The key is to get them actually wanting to eat a healthy diet and to be more active. Even the fittest children today spend significantly more time in front of some form of screen than you or I ever did, and with fears over road and personal safety, they are more likely to be driven to the school gate than to walk.

If you are concerned about your child's weight, start by getting him or her to exercise more – go walking or cycling as a family, get out in the garden with them and kick a football around – you never know, your waistline might benefit too!

MYTH BUSTERS
Let's take a look at some of the myths that we hear about obesity

I AM FAT BECAUSE I HAVE A SLOW METABOLISM	FALSE	In fact, overweight people expend more energy than thin people. Try walking around with a 10kg (22lb) backpack on all the time; you'll find that everything takes more energy. As a rough guide, the typical energy requirement for a 100kg (15st) woman to maintain her weight is 2,250kcal per day, compared to around 1,800kcal per day for a similar woman who weighs only 60kg (9st 6lb).
I AM FAT BECAUSE IT IS IN MY GENES – ALL MY FAMILY ARE FAT	FALSE	Research has shown a genetic tendency for some people to gain weight more easily than others but this isn't the whole story. Of course obesity runs in families, but much of this is due to bad eating habits and lack of exercise – nurture rather than nature.
I AM FAT BECAUSE I HAVE A PROBLEM WITH MY GLANDS	FALSE	Although medical conditions such as an underactive thyroid and polycystic ovary syndrome can be associated with weight gain, they are relatively rare and can be easily excluded by your doctor with blood tests.
I HARDLY EAT A THING ALL DAY	FALSE	It sounds cruel, but the reason for weight gain is essentially simple: you are taking in more energy than you are using. Studies have consistently shown that people who "graze" rather than eat three proper meals a day underestimate their daily energy intake by 50–80kcals per day. If you fall into this category, try keeping a food diary. Note down everything you eat for at least a week – no cheating – you must include even the three chips off your child's supper plate. You may shock yourself.

BOWEL CANCER

This is the third most common cancer in the UK, and it kills about 17,000 people each year. The sad thing is that many of these deaths could have been prevented if the disease had been detected and treated in its early stages.

WHAT ARE THE RISK FACTORS?

The main risk factors are:

• Age – bowel cancer is rare under the age of about 40.

• A family history of bowel cancer.

Most bowel cancers start as a benign polyp (growth) in the intestine. A polyp can be present for up to ten years before it turns cancerous. If the polyp is removed before this happens, your cancer risk disappears.

BOWEL CANCER SCREENING TEST

If your doctor offers you or a member of your family a screening test for bowel cancer, take it. It involves collecting three samples of your faeces, which will be analysed for minute traces of blood. If blood is detected, you will probably have further tests to confirm that it is cancer, and to discover if it has spread.

HOW IS IT TREATED?

Treatment is usually by surgery to remove the growth, which, if it is an isolated polyp, is usually curative. More advanced cases may require more extensive surgery plus chemotherapy and/or radiotherapy.

> **! SEEK MEDICAL ADVICE NOW**
> **If you notice any of the following:**
>
> • Your bowel habits change for six weeks or more.
> • There is blood in your faeces.
> • You lose weight unintentionally.
> • When you open your bowels, you feel you could go again – this is called tenesmus.
>
> Most people who have these symptoms will not have bowel cancer but they mustn't be ignored.

▾ *Consulting your doctor as soon as warning signs appear can be vital for early diagnosis and treatment of bowel cancer.*

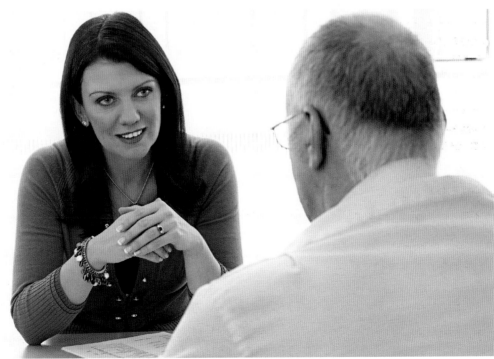

• Diabetes was first recognized as an illness 3,500 years ago • There are more than two million diabetics in the UK and experts believe that there are at least another 750,000 out there who don't yet know they have diabetes • Type 2 diabetes used to be associated with weight gain in older people, but due to the obesity epidemic we are seeing type 2 diabetes in children as young as seven • More than 80 per cent of diabetics are type 2, many of whom wouldn't be if they lost weight • Asians and Afro-caribbeans are at greater risk of type 2 diabetes.

8

Diabetes

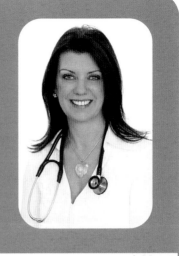

Introduction One particular organ in your body, the pancreas (which sits behind your stomach), produces a substance (hormone) called insulin, which controls the level of glucose (sugar) in your blood. You get glucose from obvious sources like sugar and sweet foods, but also from digestion of starchy foods like potatoes, pasta, rice, and bread.

Diabetes, or diabetes mellitus to give it its full name, occurs when the pancreas stops producing sufficient insulin to control the amount of sugar in the blood , or when the tissues become resistant to its effects, resulting in high blood sugar levels. Classic symptoms include weight loss, excessive thirst and fatigue, but when diabetes develops slowly the symptoms can be easily missed.

When I first qualified as a GP, it was unusual to pick up a new diagnosis of diabetes. Today, we seem to be finding new diabetics every week. The disease is one of the biggest health issues facing the UK in the 21st century, and one that is predicted to continue to increase dramatically in the next few years if we don't make lifestyle changes.

TYPES OF DIABETES

Diabetes is surprisingly common. There are over two million people in the UK with the condition and it is thought that there could be at least another 750,000 people who have it but don't yet know. There are two main types of diabetes, type 1 and type 2; the latter is by far the most common, accounting for around 85 per cent of all cases.

TYPE 1 DIABETES

This develops when the insulin-producing cells in the pancreas fail. No one really knows why this happens. It commonly starts in childhood, and those with it require lifelong insulin replacement by injection. Typical symptoms include weight loss, excessive thirst, and needing to pass lots of urine.

TYPE 2 DIABETES

In people with type 2 diabetes the pancreas still makes some insulin but not enough, or the insulin that is produced does not work properly (known as insulin resistance). Type 2 diabetes develops much more slowly than type 1 and so is much easier to miss. Most people with type 2 diabetes can be treated with lifestyle changes,

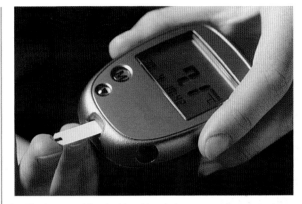

▲ Testing your blood with a blood glucose monitor gives a reading of your sugar level.

such as weight loss, a special diet, and increased exercise, although some may also need tablets. Insulin injections are not usually needed, unless the diabetes cannot otherwise be controlled.

LIVING WITH DIABETES

Being diagnosed with diabetes is a steep learning curve. You will find that you will have lots of appointments with doctors and nurses and you may feel bombarded with information. No one expects you to remember everything first time round, so don't be frightened to repeat questions or ask your nurse to write things down. It will be a bit daunting at first, but once you have your diabetes under control you should be able to lead a full and normal life, although it may take a bit more planning than previously in terms of meal times and medications.

You don't have to tell work colleagues, friends, or family, but I encourage all my patients to tell those close to them, not least so that they know what to do in an emergency (see next page). You will have to inform the DVLA and your insurance company, although having diabetes shouldn't stop you driving.

GETTING SUPPORT

There will probably be a patient support group close to you. If your surgery doesn't know of one, Diabetes UK will be able to point you in the right direction. Many of my patients have found these groups invaluable. They are a great opportunity to meet other people with diabetes, many of whom will have had a lot of the same fears and concerns as you, and may well have helpful advice.

? DID YOU KNOW

Who is at risk of type 2 diabetes?

Eight out of ten people with type 2 diabetes are overweight and weight loss could cure the problem. Other risk factors include:

- Having a big waist – a waist of over 80cm (32in) for a woman and 92cm (37in) for a man significantly increases the risk of developing diabetes.
- A family history of diabetes.
- Getting older.
- Being Asian or Afro-Caribbean.
- Developing diabetes when pregnant (gestational diabetes) – up to half of the women who have this will go on to develop the condition later in life.
- Being overweight and having polycystic ovary syndrome – around half of these women will develop diabetes by middle age.

WHAT TO DO IN AN EMERGENCY

Diabetes can cause problems if your sugar levels are either too high or too low. If you have not had enough medication or you have an infection, your sugar levels tend to run high. If you have inadvertently taken too much medication, have missed a meal, have been exercising more than usual, or have had too much alcohol, your sugar level can fall too low. If your sugar levels are too high or low, follow the advice in the box below.

ARE THERE LONG-TERM RISKS WITH DIABETES?

Unfortunately, there is a long list of possible health problems associated with diabetes. The good news is that you minimize many of them by controlling your diabetes and having regular check-ups, which can pick up any problems at an early stage and could make all the difference to your long-term health. The main long-term risks associated with diabetes are:

• Heart disease, stroke, and peripheral vascular disease.
• High blood pressure.
• Eye problems (known as retinopathy), which may cause difficulties with vision.
• Kidney disease.
• Nerve damage, which may cause anything from impotence to loss of sensation in the feet, making you more prone to ulcers as you won't feel any pain.

! EMERGENCY – DIAL 999

If your blood sugar levels fall below 4mmol/l, you will usually feel sweaty and shaky, and may notice tingling sensations. Most people with diabetes know these warning signs mean they need to eat something sugary. If you ignore these signs, you run the risk of falling into a coma. Both very high and very low sugar levels can cause unconsciousness, and you have no way of knowing which is which without checking blood sugar levels. This is a medical emergency and you should dial 999 immediately.

FIND OUT MORE
www.diabetes.org.uk

CHILDREN AND DIABETES

Like adults, children can suffer from type 1 or type 2 diabetes. Just a decade ago, I would have told you that diabetes that developed in childhood was always type 1.
In fact, type 2 diabetes was often referred to as "maturity-onset diabetes" because it was only seen in older people. Now, though, we are seeing a terrifying number of children being diagnosed with type 2 diabetes.

TYPE 1 DIABETES IN CHILDREN

Children who develop type 1 diabetes will need insulin injections. After the diagnosis, your child will probably be admitted to hospital for a few days to fine-tune the insulin dose and to give you the chance to ask the many questions you'll have. While in hospital, your child's blood sugar will be allowed to fall below normal; this is called a "hypo" and it's important that your child can recognize the signs (lightheadedness, nausea, shakiness) so he or she can take the appropriate action in future.

TYPE 2 DIABETES IN CHILDREN

Type 2 diabetes is directly linked to obesity and, as a parent, you can protect your child from developing it by watching his or her weight. If your child does develop type 2 diabetes, he or she will probably need the same treatment as adults – lifestyle changes, diet, and exercise; some children may also need medication.

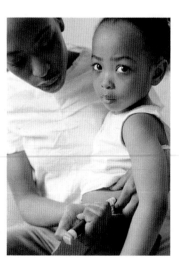

Children with type 1 diabetes will need insulin injections. ▸

MYTH BUSTERS
Like all common conditions, diabetes has myths that we should deal with.

EATING LOTS OF SWEETS CAN GIVE YOU DIABETES	FALSE	If you already have diabetes you need to watch your sugar intake, but eating sweet things won't give you diabetes.
STRESS CAN CAUSE DIABETES	FALSE	Stress can make the symptoms worse in someone who already has diabetes, but it won't cause the condition.
FEELING DIZZY IF YOU MISS A MEAL COULD BE A SIGN YOU HAVE DIABETES	FALSE	I am often asked this. If you miss a meal, your blood sugar levels fall and this can make you feel quite shaky and dizzy. However, undiagnosed diabetes actually produces the opposite problem as your sugar levels are too high.
PEOPLE WITH DIABETES SHOULDN'T EXERCISE	FALSE	Try telling that to Steve Redgrave, the Olympic rower! Exercise is good for all of us and particularly if you have diabetes as you have an increased risk of heart disease so need to try even harder at minimizing your risk factors. Routine day-to-day exercise shouldn't impact on your normal diabetes care, but if you are planning more vigorous or prolonged physical activity, you may need to fine-tune your medication and keep some carbohydrate snacks handy – ideally a combination of fast-acting carbohydrates such as glucose tablets and slow-acting ones like cereal bars. There is one important exception to this: I wouldn't advise you to exercise if your blood sugar is greater than 15mmol/l; you should get your blood sugar back under control first.

TRAVELLING WITH DIABETES

Even if your diabetes is well controlled, travelling can be difficult – mealtimes may be unpredictable and delays are always a possibility – and then there are the time differences to cope with.

TIPS TO MAKE TRAVELLING EASIER

• Carry your medication (including needles and syringes) in a clear plastic bag as hand luggage – there may be a long delay and you may need access to your insulin or tablets. Also, insulin may freeze in the hold of an aircraft and will therefore be less effective.

• To minimize security problems at airports, ask your doctor to give you a covering letter explaining why you need medication and/or needles and syringes on board, and/or carry a diabetes photo-identity card (available from Diabetes UK) that has been signed by your doctor or nurse.

• Take a copy of your prescriptions with you in case you lose your medication and need to get some more.

• Carry a combination of fast- and slow-acting carbohydrate snacks with you. This is particularly important if you are flying long-haul from east to west as the change in time zone may mean you have to put your watch back several hours, resulting in a long wait between meals.

• Every day your kidneys filter about 180 litres (320 pints) of water • Each kidney contains a million nephrons to carry out this work • The nephrons in a kidney are actually a series of complex minute tubes (tubules), which if laid end to end would stretch about 160km (100 miles) • When your bladder is full it stretches up to the level of your navel • 1 litre (1⅓ pints) of blood passes through your kidneys every minute • You can live healthily with just one kidney. In fact, you can manage without dialysis until around 90 per cent of your renal function is lost.

9

Urinary system

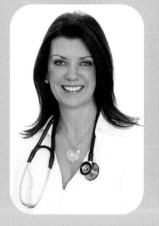

Introduction The urinary system comprises two bean-shaped kidneys, each about 12cm (5in) long, which sit on either side of your body, about half way up your abdomen towards the back. The left kidney is slightly higher than the right, which lies beneath the liver. Each kidney contains many nephrons, which are responsible for filtering blood as it passes through the kidney. The waste products that are removed from the blood are then excreted, along with water, as urine via two ureters, which connect each kidney to the bladder. Urine produced in the kidneys is stored in the bladder, ready to be excreted from the body via one tube, the urethra.

Our kidneys have other functions too. They control the composition of our blood, which is essential for the body to work properly, and play a role in fine-tuning our blood pressure via a complex system involving the secretion of enzymes and hormones. When our blood pressure falls, receptors in the kidney tubules trigger the secretion of these chemicals to increase the amount of salt and water retained by the kidneys, thereby returning blood pressure to normal. The kidneys also produce vitamin D and the hormone erythropoietin, which stimulates the production of red blood cells.

CYSTITIS

This is an inflammation of the bladder and it is often caused by a bacterial infection. It is much more common in women than men and produces symptoms that many women will be familiar with: a feeling of bursting to go to the loo only to find that you produce a tiny amount of urine that feels as if you are passing liquid razor blades. Other symptoms may include pain in the abdomen, which may radiate up to the back or down the thighs, and sometimes fever and shivering attacks.

IS CYSTITIS ALWAYS DUE TO AN INFECTION?

No, it isn't. I see a lot of postmenopausal women who suffer from mild symptoms of cystitis. Usually this isn't caused by bacterial infection at all, but occurs because the urethra (the tube that leads from the bladder to the outside world) has become inflamed from the lack of oestrogen. Another condition is "honeymoon cystitis" which is the result of vigorous sex causing inflammation, and encouraging bugs to travel up the urethra.

If you are susceptible to cystitis, symptoms can be triggered by not drinking enough fluids (dehydration), or bladder irritants such as caffeine, alcohol, or nicotine.

WHAT CAN BE DONE?

A bacterial infection will need antibiotics and if you have the classic cystitis symptoms, your doctor may be happy to talk to you on the phone and leave a prescription out for you rather than see you in the surgery.

For postmenopausal cystitis, your doctor will probably prescribe local oestrogen in the form of a cream or pessary; this is usually all that is needed to get rid of the symptoms completely.

Honeymoon cystitis usually needs antibiotics. If it is a recurrent problem you may need to adjust your love making – avoiding perfumed lubricants, and emptying your bladder after intercourse may help.

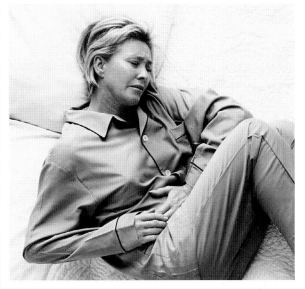

▲ Cystitis due to a bacterial infection may not only cause frequent, painful urination but also pain in the abdomen.

DR DAWN'S HEALTH CHECK
Minimizing the risk of cystitis

Recurrent urinary tract infections in women, and a single attack in men should be investigated. Talk to your doctor about having tests to check that your bladder is emptying properly and to make sure that you don't have a kidney stone. In the meantime:

• Drink plenty of fluid – at least eight large glasses a day, preferably water.

• Avoid alcohol, caffeine, and fizzy drinks because they irritate the bladder.

• Drink cranberry juice every day – if you don't like it, you can try capsules, which work just as well.

• Don't use spermicides, or condoms impregnated with spermicide, when having sex.

• Always empty your bladder after intercourse.

• Avoid perfumed soaps or bubble baths as they can alter the pH of your skin, which encourages bacterial growth.

• Wipe front to back after having a wee.

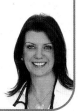

FIND OUT MORE
www.cobfoundation.org

INCONTINENCE

At least five million people in the UK report suffering from incontinence and, believe me, that is probably a gross underestimate. I wonder how many people will read this section because they have the occasional accident but have never told anyone.

TYPES OF INCONTINENCE

There are three main types of urinary incontinence:

• Stress incontinence – the type most commonly suffered by women after giving birth.
• Urge incontinence – when the bladder is irritable and contracts uncontrollably.
• Mixed incontinence – a mixture of the two types above.

STRESS INCONTINENCE

This is by far the most common form of incontinence, causing leakage of urine when we exert ourselves – anything from sneezing violently to running for a bus. For some, even stretching up to get something off a shelf will cause a leak.

Giving birth is the single greatest risk factor for incontinence, as it weakens the pelvic floor muscles. About four in ten women who have had a baby will have some incontinence; for most, it will be transient – only about one in ten women has persistent problems.

WHAT YOU CAN DO

Pelvic-floor exercises are the mainstay of treatment for stress incontinence and they solve the incontinence for three out of four women. It's never too late to start them, and you should keep them up for life. Getting them right can be difficult at first but when you know what to do, they are really simple.

If you are not sure you are doing them correctly, then ask a continence nurse or physiotherapist to show you. You can make your own appointment at the local continence clinic; you don't need to be referred by your doctor. Contact the Continence Foundation (see p.110), type in your postcode, and you'll find the address for the nearest clinic.

WHAT IF PELVIC-FLOOR EXERCISES DON'T WORK?

If pelvic-floor exercises alone don't help, it is worth seeing a continence nurse or physiotherapist, who will be able to advise on more advanced methods available. For example:

• Weighted vaginal cones – these are small cones that are held in the vagina for about 15 minutes at a time; the weight of the cones is gradually increased as the muscles become stronger.
• Electrical stimulation – this sounds terrifying but it's not. Electric probes are used to stimulate and strengthen the pelvic floor. It can give you a tingling sensation but it's not painful. Sometimes this is used to demonstrate exactly what it feels like to tighten your pelvic-floor muscles.

? DID YOU KNOW
Who is at risk

Those most at risk include women who have:

• Big babies.
• Multiple pregnancies.
• A long second stage of labour.
• An instrumental delivery (forceps or suction with a ventouse).
• An episiotomy or tear during labour.

DR DAWN'S HEALTH CHECK
Making lifestyle changes

If you suffer with an overactive bladder:

• Lose excess weight – this may be putting pressure on your bladder.
• If you smoke, stop now – nicotine irritates the bladder lining.
• Cut down on alcohol, and swap coffee and tea for decaffeinated varieties.
• Avoid fizzy drinks – these also irritate the bladder.
• Don't over restrict your fluids – concentrated urine could make the problem worse. Aim for six to eight large glasses of fluid a day (water is best).
• Some people find drinking cranberry juice also helps.

• Biofeedback – this method uses electrical signals linked to a computer to see you are doing the exercises correctly. To be honest, I don't think it works any better than exercises on their own but it can help you learn how to do the exercises properly.

OTHER TREATMENTS

There is a drug available on prescription that helps with stress incontinence. There are also various surgical treatments, ranging from injecting gel (like the one used to plump out lips) into the tissues around the urethra, or placing a tape around the neck of the bladder – both of these operations are done under local anaesthetic – to more major surgery under general anaesthetic to reposition the bladder and improve its support.

URGE INCONTINENCE

The normal bladder needs to be emptied four to eight times a day and usually gives us plenty of warning. However, if you have an overactive bladder (OAB) it may contract uncontrollably and without warning, resulting in sometimes large leaks of urine. Not surprisingly, sufferers' lives become ruled by their bladders. Many lack the confidence to move far from a toilet and often feel they have to carry spare clothes wherever they go.

There are three main types of treatment for an overactive bladder:
• Lifestyle changes (see Health check box left).
• Bladder retraining.
• Medicines.

PELVIC-FLOOR EXERCISES

Your pelvic-floor muscles are no different from any other muscles – the more you use them, the stronger they become. Before you start your exercise programme, check that you are working on the correct muscles. Sit on a chair with your legs slightly apart, then tighten your pelvic-floor muscles as if you were trying to stop yourself midstream when you are having a wee. You should feel the muscles around your anus and vagina tighten and lift. If you put a finger in your vagina, you may be able to feel the muscles squeeze your finger, although if the muscles are very weak, it will take some time to tone them up. If you are clenching your buttocks, tensing your thighs, or holding your tummy in while you do this, you are doing it wrong.

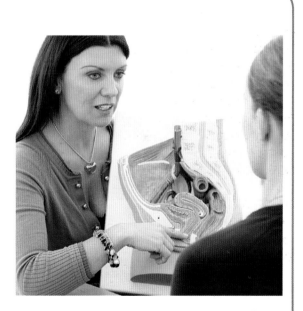

The pelvic-floor muscles support the bladder and help control the opening and closing of the bladder outlet. ▸

THE PELVIC-FLOOR WORKOUT

Once you have identified the right muscles you can move on to your pelvic-floor workout:
1 Tighten your pelvic floor and hold for a count of ten then relax for five seconds; repeat ten times if you can.
2 Tighten the muscles again but this time just for one second; repeat these rapid contractions ten times.

No-one else can see that you are doing these exercises, and if you repeat your workout several times a day you should notice a difference in four to six weeks. Try to fit it into your routine so that you don't forget them. Some of my patients say they always do them when they are waiting for a bus or standing at the school gate. After a while, you'll find yourself doing them automatically.

BLADDER RETRAINING

Start by keeping a diary for at least a week; list everything you drink, how much, and when you have it, as well as how often you pass urine. Measuring urine volume is important, so get a measuring jug and carry it everywhere that you go.

When you have completed your diary, you can set your first target – if, for example, you have been going to the toilet every hour, aim to increase the gap to 90 minutes. It may seem daunting at first, but you can make yourself "hold on" by sitting on a hard seat, doing your pelvic-floor exercises, or simply distracting yourself with something else. It can take several weeks to take effect but it can make all the difference, so stick with it.

MEDICINES

There are many different medications available to treat an overactive bladder. Talk to your doctor and don't give up if the first one doesn't suit you. Think of it like choosing clothes – one size doesn't fit all and there will be something out there for you.

▼ *Modern incontinence pads are unobtrusive and very effective, and can be invaluable if other measures have failed.*

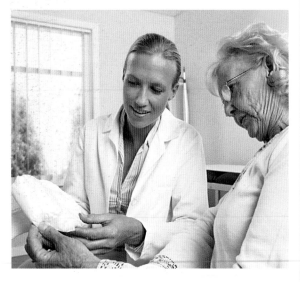

KIDNEY INFECTIONS

Most urinary tract infections are short-lived problems that are easily cleared up with a course of antibiotics and cause no lasting damage. However, infections that move up the urinary tract and into the kidney are more serious. If left untreated, such infections can cause permanent damage.

WHO IS AT RISK?

Bladder infections are usually prevented from reaching the kidney by a one-way valve at the bottom of the ureter where it enters the bladder. When the bladder contracts to empty urine, this valve shuts off, preventing urine from refluxing back up the ureter toward the kidney. In some individuals, the valve is faulty, which means that not only can urine reflux back but as soon as the bladder is emptied and relaxes, the stale urine returns to the bladder where it is even more prone to infection.

Prostate enlargement and kidney stones may also obstruct normal urine flow out of the bladder and any intervention, such as bladder surgery or the insertion of a catheter, can increase the risk of a kidney infection.

WHAT ARE THE SYMPTOMS OF A KIDNEY INFECTION?

Most kidney infections start with symptoms of cystitis – needing to wee frequently, pain on passing water (dysuria), and an urgent need to empty the bladder. As the infection takes hold, patients develop back, loin, or groin pain, a high fever, nausea, and vomiting. Some people also notice pus in their urine.

WHAT CAN BE DONE?

A urine test will be taken and if infection is confirmed, antibiotics will be prescribed. You must take the full course to make sure the infection is eradicated. Once the infection has been treated, your doctor will probably recommend that you have further tests to check if there has been any scaring or kidney damage. These tests may include an ultrasound or a special X-ray test in which dye is injected into the arm and then a series of X-rays are taken of the kidneys as the dye is excreted.

BLADDER CANCER

This affects one in every 5,000 adults in the UK and is the fourth most common cancer in men and the ninth most common cancer in women. Smoking and exposure to certain industrial chemicals may increase your risk of developing bladder cancer.

WHAT ARE THE SYMPTOMS?

Bladder cancer may not cause symptoms in its early stages. The first indications are typically blood in the urine (without being accompanied by pain) or recurrent urinary tract infections. If you notice either, see your doctor to get them checked out.

CAN IT BE TREATED?

Thankfully, most bladder cancers are very slow-growing. About eight out of ten cancers can be removed with diathermy (heat treatment) carried out using a special instrument called a cystoscope, and don't usually need any further treatment.

REDUCING YOUR RISK

• Stop smoking – some of the cancer-causing chemicals in cigarette smoke are absorbed into the bloodstream and then filtered out and excreted in the urine. Long term, the presence of these chemicals in the urine increases the risk of bladder cancer. Stopping smoking reduces the risk not only of developing bladder cancer but also of it recurring.

• Take appropriate precautions if you work in the rubber, paint, dye, printing, or textile industries. Workers in these industries are at increased risk. Your employer will advise you about protective clothing.

• Avoid swimming in ponds, streams, or canals in tropical countries. These waters are often home to a particular snail that harbours a parasite which causes bilharzia in humans – a condition associated with an increased risk of bladder cancer.

• Eat five portions of fruit and vegetables a day, and keep to a low-fat diet.

KIDNEY CANCER

Kidney cancer is not very common. It occurs twice as often in men as in women and two out of three patients are aged over 65.

TREATMENT AND REDUCING YOUR RISK

Kidney cancer is treated by removing the affected kidney (the other can compensate), which is often all the treatment needed. You can reduce your risk of developing it by:

• Stopping smoking – smoking doubles your risk.

• Watching your weight – a BMI greater than 30 increases your risk.

• Getting your blood pressure treated if it is high, as it is associated with an increased risk of kidney cancer.

• Taking appropriate precautions at work – people in the dry-cleaning, steel, or petrochemical industries and those working with asbestos could all be at higher risk of developing kidney cancer.

▼ *An X-ray revealing a kidney tumour (bright white area).*

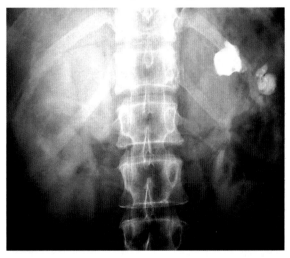

> **!** **SEEK MEDICAL ADVICE NOW**
> **If you have any combination of:**
> • Blood in your urine.
> • Pain in your loin.
> • Night sweats.
> • A lump in your abdomen.

• An average adult skeleton has 206 bones • The largest bone is the thigh bone and the smallest is the minute stirrup bone that sits behind the eardrum and is only about 3mm (1/10 in) long • Most of the body's red blood cells are formed in the bone marrow, the soft fatty substance that fills the cavities in your bones; most of the marrow is made in your thigh bones • Children replace their entire skeleton with new bone every two years! As we age, that rapid turnover of bone slows down.

10

Bones

Introduction The skeleton is an amazing structure. It supports your body and surrounds and protects the key organs, like your heart, lungs, liver, and brain. Yet most of us don't give our bones a second thought, not until we break one that is. Most people think of bones as being static. In fact nothing could be further from the truth – bone is alive and constantly changing. Bones have a hard outer casing, and a cavity in the centre, which is filled with a substance called bone marrow.

Your bones stop growing in length by your late teens or early twenties, but they continue to develop in strength until your mid-twenties, when you reach what's called your peak bone mass. Although your bone is still being broken down and rebuilt up at this point, the total amount stays the same. After the age of about 35, your bone begins to be broken down slightly faster than your body can build it up again. As a result your skeleton actually starts to become thinner as part of the natural ageing process.

Bones are held together at their joints by bands of elastic tissue called ligaments, while muscles are attached to the bones by tendons. Movement is created by muscles, which work in pairs – one contracts while the other relaxes, thereby pulling the bones away from and towards each other.

FROZEN SHOULDER

The term "frozen shoulder" encompasses a number of conditions that cause a stiff, painful shoulder with restricted movement. It occurs most commonly in middle age or later life and often follows a minor injury.

WHAT YOU CAN DO

Usually people come to see me in the surgery because they are fed up with being unable to do up a bra or reach back to brush their hair. The important thing is to get the joint mobile again. Anti-inflammatory medicines will help. Placing a hot pad on your shoulder 20 minutes before you exercise can increase muscle movement by up to 20 per cent.

MEDICAL ADVICE

A physiotherapist will be able to advise you on a suitable exercise programme. If you are still struggling, talk to your doctor about having a steroid injection into the joint. He or she may refer you to a specialist for this.

▾ Joint mobilization is essential for treating frozen shoulder.

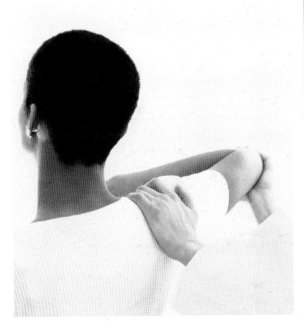

RESTLESS LEG SYNDROME

As many as one in ten people suffers from legs that twitch and jerk when they are tired in the evenings. It is particularly common during pregnancy but can also be associated with low iron levels and kidney disease.

WHAT YOU CAN DO

Some medications, including antidepressants, antihistamines, and some blood pressure treatments, can make it worse. If you are taking any of these, it is worth talking to your doctor to see if a change in medication would help.

I often find that some simple lifestyle changes are all that is needed. Numerous treatments have been tried over the years, including tranquilizers, painkillers, and antiepileptic drugs, but none of them are licensed for treating restless legs in this country.

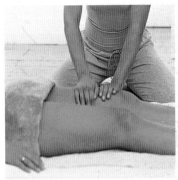

Leg massage may help relieve the symptoms of restless leg syndrome. ▸

DR DAWN'S HEALTH CHECK
Preventing restless leg syndrome

The following tips can either prevent restless legs or help when you are suffering from them:

- Establish a regular bedtime routine, going to bed and getting up at the same time each day.
- Avoid catnapping during the day.
- Cut down on your alcohol.
- Reduce your caffeine intake and avoid it altogether after six in the evening.
- If you are a smoker, give it up.
- Take a relaxing bath before retiring to bed.
- Try gently massaging your legs.

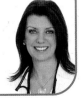

OSTEOPOROSIS

Also called brittle bone disease, this simply means thin bones, and it affects around three million people in this country. It is not a painful condition. The pain only comes when you break an affected bone. People often get osteoarthritis, which affects the joints (see p.118) which is often confused with osteoporosis, a disease of bone.

HOW WOULD I KNOW IF I HAD OSTEOPOROSIS?

Osteoporosis has no symptoms – it's a painless condition. You can have exceptionally thin bones and no warning signs of pain or morning stiffness. In fact, people usually only discover they have the condition when they have a relatively minor fall and end up in hospital with a broken bone.

It can only be reliably diagnosed with a special scan called a DEXA scan, which is a simple procedure. Unfortunately, availability of DEXA scanning varies hugely across the country. If you think you could be at risk, talk to your doctor. You may be eligible for a scan on the NHS, but if you are not and you are still concerned, it is worth considering paying for a private scan. Plain X-rays will not show osteoporosis until the disease is in very

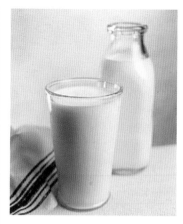

◄ *A diet rich in calcium is important for protecting against osteoporosis.*

advanced stages. Heel ultrasounds are a good in-between option – they are not as accurate as DEXA scans but they are better than nothing.

IS OSTEOPOROSIS A SERIOUS CONDITION?

Yes! There are over 70,000 osteoporotic hip fractures in the UK each year and six months after breaking a hip, one in two women are still unable to carry out basic tasks

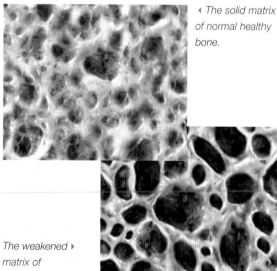

◄ *The solid matrix of normal healthy bone.*

The weakened ▶ matrix of osteoporotic bone.

? DID YOU KNOW

Who is at risk?

Many groups of people are at risk of osteoporosis. Risk factors include:

- Having a first-degree relative with osteoporosis.
- Being Caucasian or Asian.
- Being a smoker.
- Drinking alcohol beyond recommended limits.
- Taking no weight-bearing exercise.
- Having a low body weight for your height.
- Having an early menopause.
- Having your ovaries removed.
- Taking steroids.
- Stopping your periods for six months or more (excluding pregnancy) – anorexia and over-exercising will do this.
- There are also some medical conditions that make people more prone to osteoporosis, such as thyroid disease, rheumatoid arthritis, and any bowel condition that affects the absorption of nutrients such as calcium that are essential for healthy bones.

like dressing themselves. In fact, one in five will die within a year as a result of the fracture – don't leave it too late, start thinking about your bones now.

WHAT ABOUT HRT AND OSTEOPOROSIS?

Oestrogen keeps our bones strong and there is no doubt that HRT is effective at protecting against thinning of our bones, but it is not without its risks and is no longer recommended as first-line treatment for osteoporosis. However, if a woman requires HRT to control her menopausal symptoms, it will protect her bones at the same time.

IS THERE A CURE FOR OSTEOPOROSIS?

When it comes to osteoporosis, prevention really is better than cure. There are treatments to help halt bone loss and there is some evidence that they also promote new bone formation, but they will only rebuild bone at a rate of 2–3 per cent over a two-year period. That's certainly

better than nothing, but it isn't a cure and there are no short cuts – you will have to do your bit to look after your bones too. Your doctor will be able to advise you as to which treatment is best for you – some need to be taken every day, while others can be taken weekly or monthly.

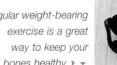

Regular weight-bearing exercise is a great way to keep your bones healthy. ▶ ▼

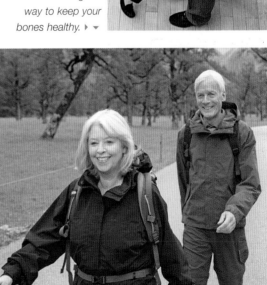

DR DAWN'S HEALTH CHECK
How you can protect your bones

Start thinking about your bone health sooner rather than later, particularly if you fall into one of the at-risk groups (see left). Begin by taking the following simple measures:

- Eat a diet rich in calcium.
- Take regular weight-bearing exercise – walking, dancing, and jogging are all excellent for maintaining healthy bones, but swimming (although good for the rest of your body) won't help strengthen your bones.
- Maintain a healthy body weight.
- If you smoke, stop now.
- Keep to the recommended daily limits for alcohol.
- Avoid fizzy drinks – they interfere with the absorption of calcium.
- If you have to take steroids for a medical condition, ask your doctor if you should be taking anything to protect your bones as well. There are lots of different treatments available to help build up your bones again. Some are taken every day, some once a week – your doctor can advise on which is the most appropriate for you.

FIND OUT MORE
www.nos.org.uk

OSTEOARTHRITIS

Also called OA, this simply means inflammation of the joints. Osteoarthritis primarily affects weight-bearing joints in the hips and knees. We can all expect to develop some wear and tear as we get older – about one and half million people in the UK receive treatment for osteoarthritis from their doctor – but that is only the tip of the iceberg, as many more sufferers self-medicate.

WHO IS AT RISK?

It is estimated that there could be as many as ten million people in the UK suffering from osteoarthritis. Your risk of developing it increases with age, especially if you have a family history of osteoarthritis or if you have injured a joint in the past.

WHAT ARE THE SYMPTOMS?

The knees, hips, hands, ankles, feet, and spine are the most commonly affected joints. Typical symptoms include pain and stiffness, particularly in the morning, and swelling and creaking in the affected joint. Symptoms are often worse in cold, damp weather.

WHAT YOU CAN DO

There is no cure for osteoarthritis, but you can ease the pain with simple painkillers – paracetamol is effective if taken regularly. Anti-inflammatory tablets also help.

If you have osteoarthritis, it is important to keep as active as you can. People always worry about making pain and stiffness worse with exercise, but keeping active will actually reduce it, particularly in the hip and knee. It can be difficult to exercise if you are in pain but the less active you are, the more likely you are to gain weight, putting extra strain on your joints. Swimming is an excellent option as it helps flexibility and, because you float in the water, you are not straining your joints.

WHAT ABOUT OTHER REMEDIES?

There is some controversy over whether or not taking the supplement glucosamine helps your joints, but I am generally in favour. All the research is based on patients taking 1500mg daily, so if you are going to try it, it makes

sense to do the same. Cod-liver oil and extract of rose hip are also worth a try, and omega-3 oils, found in oily fish such as salmon, mackerel, trout, and sardines, are great for maintaining healthy joints.

◀ X-ray of a healthy knee joint.

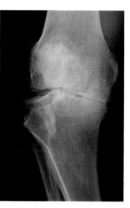

X-ray of a knee joint ▶
with osteoarthritis.

RHEUMATOID ARTHRITIS

Also called RA, this is a progressive and disabling autoimmune disease (in which the body develops antibodies to parts of itself and attacks them). In RA, the antibodies are directed at the joints, where they cause swelling and damage to the surrounding cartilage and bone. Any joint may be affected but RA most commonly affects the hands, feet, and wrists.

HOW CAN I TELL THE DIFFERENCE BETWEEN RA AND OA?

Rheumatoid arthritis often runs in families and occurs at a younger age than osteoarthritis – the first symptoms usually start between the ages of 30 and 40. Any form of arthritis can wear you down and leave you feeling tired, but rheumatoid arthritis patients feel completely exhausted and may also have a fever.

HOW IS RA TREATED?

Unfortunately, there is no cure for RA (although, with an increasing understanding of how the disease develops, we are getting closer) so treatment is aimed at controlling the symptoms. In the past, disease-modifying drugs such as methotrexate were reserved for the later stages of severe RA. It is now widely accepted that starting them earlier, and at higher doses, can improve the long-term outcome. They can have side effects but if your doctor suggests taking them, he or she will make sure you are closely monitored. Many patients find that they make all the difference to maintaining their independence.

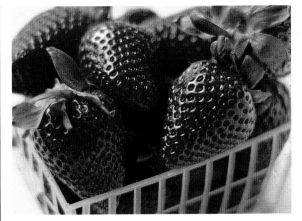

▲ Strawberries help to relieve the pain of gout in some people.

GOUT

"Grout", as my father-in-law aptly calls it, is said to be the curse of too much high living. Certainly being overweight, eating steak, and drinking red wine raise your chances of having an attack. But you don't have to lead the high life to be at risk. Gout is much more common in men than women, and if you have had one attack you're at risk of another.

CAUSES AND SYMPTOMS

Gout can develop if there is a build-up of a chemical called uric acid in your body. You take in uric acid in your diet and it's also produced during the natural turnover of your body cells. Normally, any excess is excreted in your urine but people with gout retain higher than normal levels of uric acid.

In most sufferers, symptoms flare up periodically, with the affected joint becoming red, swollen, and extremely painful. The most common site is the big toe, although any joint can be affected, and the wrist and ankle are other common sites.

HOW IS IT TREATED?

Treatment involves rest, elevation of the affected limb, taking anti-inflammatory medication, and drinking plenty

of water. You can avoid attacks by eating small, regular meals, cutting down on alcohol, avoiding high-purine foods, and drinking plenty of water. If you have frequent attacks of gout, talk to your doctor as he or she can prescribe medication that you can take every day to prevent attacks.

FOODS TO AVOID

- Meat – red meat, liver, and offal.
- Fish and shellfish – sardines, mackerel, anchovies, herrings, and fish roe.
- Spinach, asparagus, cauliflower, and mushrooms and yeast extracts.
- All alcohol, but particularly beer and red wine.

? **DID YOU KNOW**
Who is at risk?

You are at greater risk of gout if you:
- Have a family history of gout.
- Are overweight.
- Overeat or starve yourself – either can precipitate an attack.
- Drink too much alcohol.
- Have psoriasis or a blood disorder in which your body cells turn over more rapidly.
- Have a diet rich in high-purine foods.
- Are on diuretics (to prevent water retention) – don't stop prescribed medicine without talking to your doctor.

BACK PAIN

Most back pain is caused by muscle or ligament injury, and nine out of ten cases get better within six weeks, whatever you do. In the past, doctors advised anyone with back pain to take to their bed and rest. We now know that staying as active as possible is vital. Too much rest weakens your back muscles and can lengthen your recovery.

HOW THE BACK WORKS

Your back is supported by your spine, a column of 24 small bones (vertebrae), each vertabra is separated by a small "cushion" known as a disc, allowing the spine to bend. The spinal cord, a cable of nerves, runs from the brain down through this column, carrying nerve signals to the rest of your body. Damage to the spinal cord can result in serious long-term disability.

TREATING BACK PAIN

Following the initial injury – in what's referred to as the acute phase – simple painkillers, such as paracetamol, and anti-inflammatory medication will help.

The role of physiotherapy, osteopathy, and chiropractic manipulation in helping back pain is a source of debate, and I have seen all of them work. The important thing is to find a practitioner you trust and stick with him or her – it can take several treatments to get you back on track.

▼ *Physiotherapy, osteopathy, and chiropractic manipulation can be useful in overcoming back pain.*

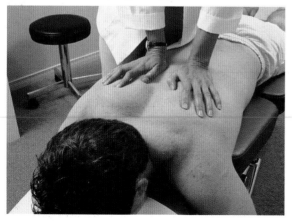

CAN SURGERY HELP?

Unless it is essential, I would advise against referral to an orthopaedic specialist. Back surgery is fraught with difficulties and so shouldn't be undertaken lightly. Of course, some people have no option but to consider surgery, and for many it is the answer.

PROTECTING YOUR BACK IN THE FUTURE

Anyone who has suffered one episode of back pain is at risk of another one. You will need to look after your back, particularly when you are lifting.

- Always bend from your knees not your back.
- Keep your feet wide apart and your back upright.
- Keep the object close to you.
- Avoid twisting and bending at the same time.

If you spend a lot of time sitting at a desk, make sure that you sit upright with your feet flat on the floor. Ideally, you should use a chair that supports your lower back.

WHAT IS A SLIPPED DISC?

Between each vertebra is a "squashy" intervertebral disc, which acts like a shock absorber and allows the spine to flex. It is said to be "slipped" when part of it bulges out of its capsule. This can press on the nerves where they come out from the spinal cord, causing severe pain in your legs and possibly weakness or numbness. In serious cases, this can cause numbness around your perineum and interfere with bladder or bowel function; this is an emergency, and surgery may be essential.

! **SEEK MEDICAL ADVICE NOW**
If you experience any of the following, as it could indicate a serious problem:

- Your pain follows an accident.
- You have any associated numbness or tingling.
- You have difficulty passing water.
- You are under 20 or over 55 with a new episode of pain.
- You or your family have a history of cancer.
- Your pain is not controlled by pain-relief medication, or it's getting worse over a period of weeks.
- You think you may have lost height.

TOP FIVE EXERCISES FOR A STRONGER BACK

Back bend ▸
Stand upright, lifting your arms up above your head. Gently lean backwards and hold for ten seconds. Repeat ten times.

Back stretch ▸
Lie on your front with your arms bent and your palms down by your shoulders. Gently push yourself up, leaving a little bend at the elbow, and hold for ten seconds. Repeat ten times.

Cat stretch ▸
Get on the floor on all fours, tighten your abdominal muscles, and slowly let your back dip toward the floor. Then tuck your bottom under, let your head drop to the floor, and arch your back up to the ceiling. Repeat five times.

Rocking knee squeezes ▸
Lie on your back on the floor, bring your knees as close to your chest as feels comfortable, then hug them. Slowly rock your knees from side to side ten times.

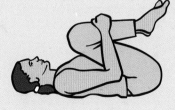

Forward arm stretch ▸
Kneel on the floor with your bottom resting on your heels and place your hands on the floor in front of you. Stretch forward as far as you can and hold for 30 seconds.

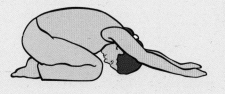

- There are 27 bones in each hand. In fact, more than half the bones in your body are found in your hands and feet
- Your hands and feet are the first to grow during your teenage growth spurt • Fingernails grow nearly four times faster than toenails. It takes around eight months to totally regrow a fingernail • The hand that you favour as a 10-week-old fetus is the one that you will favour for the rest of your life
- Two identical fingerprints have never been found – even identical twins have different fingerprints.

11

Hands

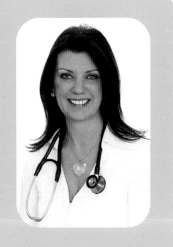

Introduction What differentiates humans and primates from other mammals, is the ability to oppose our thumbs. This means we are able to fold our thumbs inwards towards the palm of the hand and the other fingertips. It is this movement that gives us the unique ability to hold delicate objects, operate machinery, and play musical instruments.

The movements of the hand are controlled by two groups of muscles – the extrinsic and intrinsic muscle groups. The extrinsic muscles extend into the forearm and are responsible for flexing and extending the fingers. The intrinsic muscles lie within the hand and control much of the movement of the thumb and little finger.

Our fingertips have more nerve endings per square centimetre than almost anywhere else in the body, making them exceptionally sensitive to touch, pain, and temperature.

FINGERNAILS AND DISEASE

Our fingernails grow at around 0.1mm (0.004in) a day but they stop growing if you become seriously ill. When you recover, they start to grow again but this leaves a horizontal ridge. By measuring the distance from the cuticle to the ridge it is possible to date an illness with surprising accuracy.

FINGERNAILS ARE HEALTH INDICATORS

There are lots of other ways your fingernails can give away clues to your health:

• Spoon-shaped fingernails (koilonychia) may be the result of low iron levels and anaemia (see p.61) or, more seriously, a sign of angina (see p.51).

• Flaky fingernails that lift off the nail bed (onycholysis) may be due to a fungal infection or may be associated with an overactive thyroid gland or psoriasis (see p.36).

• Very pale or white fingernails may be another sign of anaemia.

• Blue-grey fingernails may be an indication of heart or lung disease.

• If you place your thumbnails together face to face, you will see a diamond-shaped space between the nail and the nail bed. If this is absent, we say someone has "clubbed" fingernails. Some people are born this way, but if clubbing develops in later life it can indicate a serious illness, such as lung, liver, or heart disease.

▼ *The shape, colour, and texture of your fingernails can be indicators of your underlying health.*

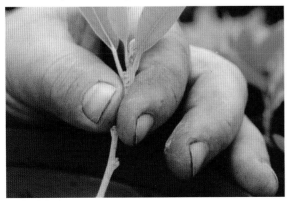

HYGIENE

Washing your hands really does make a difference. Most coughs, colds, and stomach upsets are transmitted from person to person via the hands, so washing before eating and after every visit to the toilet reduces your risk of contracting these illnesses. All you need are soap and water.

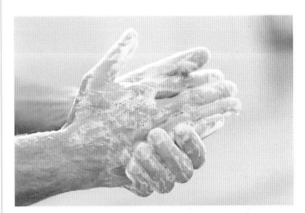

▲ *Thoroughly washing your hands with soap and water can reduce your risk of catching and spreading infections.*

WHAT ABOUT MRSA?

This is a serious bacterial infection that is resistant to many antibiotics. I am often asked about the risks of MRSA (or methicillin-resistant *Staphylococcus aureus*, to give it its full name) by patients and their relatives when they are due for an operation. There is no doubt that many of us carry the MRSA bacteria in our noses and on our hands, and although we don't seem to have any adverse effects from the bacteria when we are fit and well, if you are undergoing surgery you are at risk of infection in the wound.

REDUCING INFECTION

MRSA is transmitted by touch, and washing your hands dramatically reduces the likelihood of passing on the infection. Probably the most important thing you can do for anyone you know who is having an operation is to make sure that nobody touches them without first cleaning their hands, either by washing them with soap and water or by using an alcohol-based hand rub.

REPETITIVE STRAIN INJURY

Also known as RSI, this condition occurs when repetitive movements of the same muscles strain them, making them sore and swollen. The most common site of RSI that I see is the wrists, particularly in keyboard workers. When you press the swollen area, you can often feel a crackling; this is due to the fluid that has collected around the tendon sheath as a result of the inflammation.

WHAT YOU CAN DO

Unfortunately, there are no quick fixes. As inconvenient as it may be, you will have to stop the repetitive movement that caused the inflammation and rest the affected tendons to allow the inflammation to settle down. Anti-inflammatory medication will help, but you also still need to stop doing the things that caused the problem. When you return to work, you will need to reassess your working environment.

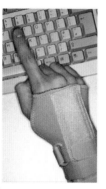

▲ A wrist splint may help relieve RSI symptoms.

DR DAWN'S HEALTH CHECK
Preventing another attack

If you have suffered with RSI and are going back to work, make sure that you:

• Take a break every hour or so and stretch your arms, fingers, and wrists.

• Split your work up whenever you can so that you don't spend long periods doing the same task.

• Adjust the height of your chair and desk so that when you are typing your forearms are at 90 degrees to your upper arms.

• Learn to touch-type properly, if you can, so that you can work in a more upright position.

• Using a gel wrist and hand support for your keyboard and computer mouse can also help.

• If you have an occupational health specialist at your workplace, ask him or her to check your workspace.

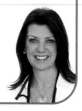

CARPAL TUNNEL SYNDROME

The carpal tunnel is a channel on the inner (flexor) surface of your wrist. This channel is bound on either side by the base of your arm bones and a tough fibrous band. A nerve (called the median nerve) that supplies sensation to your thumb, index finger, middle finger, and part of your ring finger runs through the tunnel. If there is any inflammation or swelling in the wrist joint, the median nerve is compressed.

WHAT ARE THE SYMPTOMS?

Compression of the median nerve may cause the fingers it supplies to become numb or tingle. Often, the symptoms are worse at night and, if left untreated, may develop into pain and long-term nerve damage.

WHAT CAUSES IT?

Anything that causes restriction in the tunnel may lead to carpal tunnel syndrome; common causes include:

• Pregnancy, although the symptoms usually disappear after the baby is born.

• Injury or repetitive strain injury (RSI).

• Obesity (see p.94).

• Diabetes (see p.101).

• Underactivity of the thyroid gland.

• Rheumatoid arthritis (see p.118).

WHAT YOU CAN DO

Often, all you need to do is rest the wrist. Wearing a wrist splint (especially at night) may help. A splint prevents you from bending your hand forward, an action that further restricts the space in the tunnel. Your doctor can advise you on where to get a splint fitted. Anti-inflammatory drugs, such as ibuprofen, also help, and your doctor may prescribe tablets that prevent water retention (diuretics).

If symptoms persist despite these measures, I usually recommend to patients that they have a steroid injection into the wrist space. If they are still suffering from symptoms after three steroid injections, then I refer them to an orthopaedic surgeon for an operation to release the pressure on the nerve.

RAYNAUD'S DISEASE

In this condition, exposure to cold causes small blood vessels that supply the fingers and toes (and, less commonly, the ears and nose) to go into spasm, restricting blood flow to those areas. As a result, the affected areas become pale, then blue, and finally bright red. In severe cases, spasm of the blood vessels may be triggered simply by touching a cold object or by stress. Raynaud's affects about ten million people in the UK, 90 per cent of whom are women.

WHAT YOU CAN DO

• Don't smoke – smoking lowers your body temperature by as much as one degree.

• Wear extra pairs of gloves and/or socks in cold weather.

• Warm your socks and gloves before wearing them.

• Have warm drinks regularly to keep your hands warm.

• Buy a thermal pocket handwarmer and/or shoe inserts.

• Avoid carrying heavy bags in your hand – these can obstruct the circulation. Use a shoulder bag instead.

• The herbal remedy ginkgo biloba improves circulation; many of my patients have found it helps their Raynaud's.

If these measures don't work, talk to your doctor about prescription drugs to improve circulation.

▼ Wearing gloves to keep your hands warm prevents symptoms of Raynaud's.

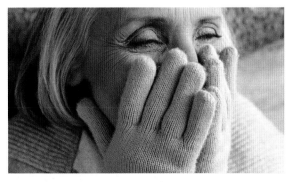

FIND OUT MORE
www.raynauds.org.uk

GANGLION

A ganglion is a fluid-filled cyst that often develops near joints, usually around the wrist or on the inner (palmar) surface of the fingers. Ganglions are the most common cause of swellings in the hand.

CAN YOU REALLY HIT A GANGLION WITH A HEAVY BOOK TO GET RID OF IT?

Yes – hitting a ganglion simply causes the cyst to rupture. However, although this is effective, the cyst often forms again. A ganglion is harmless and almost always painless, but if any of my patients is really bothered by a ganglion, I refer them to an orthopaedic surgeon who can remove the cyst, but even then up to one in five recurs.

▼ A ganglion is a harmless, fluid-filled cyst that often develops on the wrist.

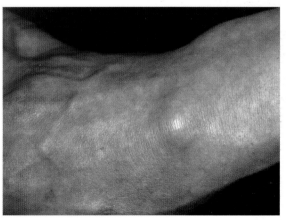

? DID YOU KNOW
Right-handedness

Around 90 per cent of us are right-handed. The only other species known to show such a consistent bias is the parrot – 90 per cent of them choose to use their left foot when picking something up! And it's not just our hands, most of us are also right-footed. This dominance of one side is reflected in the brain: in right-handed people, the brain's left side is dominant and vice versa.

• There are 26 bones in each foot • The skin on the sole of the feet (and on the palms of the hands) contains no pigment cells and so will not tan • It takes 12–18 months to regrow a toenail • Like fingerprints, foot prints are unique to each individual and start to develop at about 13 weeks after conception • The average human step is about 70cm (28in) long.

12

Feet

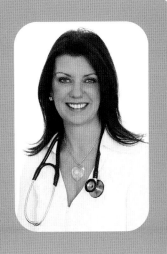

Introduction We take very little notice of our feet until they smell or hurt. Feet are complex structures of bones, muscles, and ligaments that keep us both upright and mobile. Without them we are grounded.

The bones in our feet are arranged in three arches – two run lengthways, and one runs across the foot. It is these arches that give our feet their strength and stability. Tough ligaments bind the bones together but also allow for some movement. Most of our weight is carried through just two bones in the heel called the calcaneus and the talus, and most of the movement of the foot is achieved by contraction and relaxation of muscles in the lower leg rather than the foot itself.

Our feet are a relatively small base on which we stand. Constant messages between the muscles of our feet and our brains allow for minute movements to ensure that we stay in balance. In fact, we rely heavily on our big toes for our posture – people who have had to have their big toe amputated can take a long time learning to walk again.

ATHLETE'S FOOT

This is a very common fungal infection that affects as many as one in six adults. Its name comes from the fact that fungi thrive in warm sweaty environments – trainers are a fungus's paradise.

WHAT YOU CAN DO

There are several antifungal creams and ointments available over the counter from your chemist. They all work but the most effective contain a substance called terbinafine – ask your pharmacist for advice. Very occasionally, doctors prescribe antifungal tablets for severe athlete's foot that doesn't respond to creams, but I avoid it if I can as these tablets have lots of side effects.

TIPS FOR KEEPING ATHLETE'S FOOT IN CHECK

• Wash your feet every day and dry them well – take special care between your toes.
• Spend as much time as you can barefoot.
• Avoid wearing trainers whenever possible.
• Sweaty shoes can take 24–48 hours to dry out. Try not to wear the same shoes all the time; if that's not possible, dry your shoes on a low setting with a hair dryer.
• Avoid perfumed products – these can change the pH of your skin, which encourages the fungus to grow.
• Use a dusting powder in your shoes to prevent athlete's foot – they aren't as effective as treatments for athlete's foot but regular use may prevent recurrences.
• If you get athlete's foot repeatedly, ask your doctor to test you for diabetes – resistant fungal infections may be a sign that your sugar levels are too high.

▾ *Athlete's foot causes itchy, flaky, sore areas of skin, most commonly between the toes.*

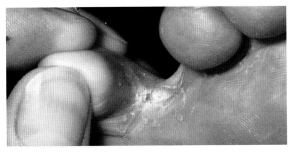

INGROWING TOENAIL

If a toenail is ingrowing, it means that it's curving or growing into the skin on one or both sides of the nail. Anyone who has had an ingrowing toenail will tell you that it is excruciatingly painful and literally stops you in your tracks. They are, however, relatively easy to prevent.

WHEN TO SEE YOUR DOCTOR

You should see your doctor as soon as you notice any redness, particularly if it's very painful, because it's possible it may be infected. Your doctor may prescribe antibiotics for an infection and may recommend that you see a chiropodist. If you repeatedly suffer from an ingrowing toenail, your doctor may suggest an operation to remove part or all of the nail.

PREVENTING INGROWING TOENAILS

• Always cut your toenails straight across.
• Avoid cutting your toenails too short – you should be able to see the nail above the skin.
• If you have suffered from ingrowing toenails before, try soaking your feet for a few minutes and, when the nail is soft, place a tiny wedge of cotton wool under each side to encourage the nail to grow upwards rather than down.

▾ *Toenails should be cut straight across and not too short (left) not shaped and below the end of the toe (right).*

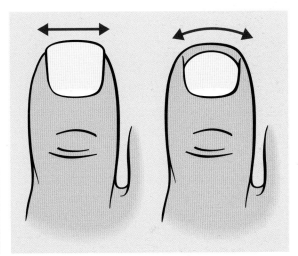

BUNIONS

You will be familiar with the unsightly swelling, or deformity, that can develop at the base of the big toe. You will probably call it a bunion, but doctors call it a hallux valgus. They are extremely common, particularly in women over the age of 50, but I have seen them in much younger people.

DO HIGH HEELS CAUSE BUNIONS?

Probably not. At least not on their own, but before you rush out to buy another pair of stilettos, they play their part. The single greatest risk for developing a bunion is a family history: at least two-thirds of all those who have bunions will have another member of the family with the same problem. In societies that go around barefoot, bunions are almost unheard of, so it's reasonable to assume that footwear may play a role. Believe me, at 163cm (5ft 4in) I like my heels. But if your mother had bunions you could too, so it's worth being sensible about your shoes.

CAN I STOP MY BUNIONS GETTING WORSE?

While high heels are not necessarily the sole cause of bunions, it makes sense to swap your elegant shoes for well-fitting, more sensible footwear. Chiropodists often recommend exercises that strengthen the muscles and tendons around your big toe. Here's one you can try. Put your feet side by side, and try to move your big toes towards each other. Do this three or four times a day, while you're in the bath or in bed.

WHEN SHOULD I CONSIDER SURGERY?

The short answer is: when your bunions hurt. By the time the toe has bent inwards by 30 degrees or more, the deformity is irreversible without surgery, but even then I still wouldn't advise rushing into an operation. Bunion surgery has come a long way in the last decade or so, but it is still quite a major undertaking and you will be off your feet for several weeks. For this reason, it shouldn't be considered for cosmetic reasons alone, and surgery should definitely be avoided in teenagers because they tend to have a high recurrence rate – as much as 40 per cent.

CHILBLAINS

These are red itchy patches most commonly found on the tops of the toes (and fingers). They form in cold weather, but actually it's not so much the temperature as the degree of humidity that seems to be the trigger – cold, damp conditions cause the most problems. This is why, for example, chilblains are common in Britain but rarely seen in the Arctic. Around one in ten UK adults suffers from chilblains, most of them women.

WHAT YOU CAN DO

Here are my top tips to avoiding chilblains:
- Don't smoke – smoking reduces the body temperature by as much as one degree and impairs circulation.
- Avoid wearing tightly fitting shoes.
- Wear extra pairs of socks – several thin pairs will be better than thick ones that can make your shoes too tight and impede circulation.
- Get foot warmers for your shoes.
- Keep moving – exercise improves circulation.
- Warm your feet or massage them when you come in from the cold to improve the blood flow.
- Don't scratch your chilblains – you run the risk of breaking the skin and developing an infection.
- Try alternating hot and cold footbaths – three minutes in warm water, 30 seconds in cold, to stimulate the circulation in the toes.

▼ *Chilblains are red, itchy areas that usually affect the tops of the toes and sometimes the fingers.*

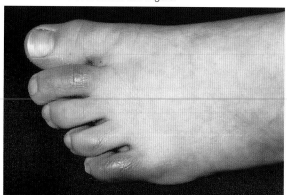

PLANTAR FASCIITIS

Caused by inflammation of the broad fibrous band (called the plantar fascia) that supports the base of the foot, plantar fasciitis is the most common cause of pain in the heel. It may also sometimes cause pain in the arch of the foot.

WHAT CAUSES IT?

- Abnormalities of the arch of the foot – flat feet and high-arched feet can both cause problems.
- Obesity, because the extra weight puts extra pressure on your heels.
- Increased exercise, particularly running on hard surfaces.
- Badly fitting shoes, especially high heels.

WHAT YOU CAN DO

The good news is that most cases clear up within about a year regardless of what you do, but here are some tips on how to help speed your recovery:

- If you are overweight, lose the excess weight.
- Wear soft shoes with good arch support.
- Rest your foot when you can.
- Avoid running on hard or uneven surfaces.
- Try some foot-stretching exercises – roll the arch of your foot forward and back over a cylindrical tin (such as a tin of food) to stretch the plantar fascia. Stretching the calf muscles will also help.
- Try taking an over-the-counter anti-inflammatory drug, such as ibuprofen.
- Consider putting a heel support or an arch support in your shoes. Alternatively, you could try special orthotic insoles; available from some sport shops, these are shaped to support all parts of your feet, and some are available that can be moulded to your individual feet.

WHEN SHOULD YOU SEEK MEDICAL ADVICE?

If you are still suffering despite these measures, then talk to your doctor. He or she may suggest a steroid injection, which can be effective in the short term, but they are not suitable for everyone. Some doctors will do this in their surgery but success does depend on how accurately the injection is given. Doctors who do not do this regularly may prefer to refer you to a specialist. In extreme cases,

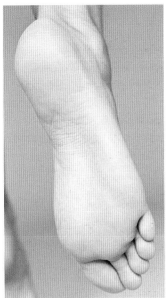

Plantar fasciitis is caused by inflammation of the broad band of fibrous tissue that runs from the heel to the toes and supports the base of the foot. ▸

there is an operation that can relieve the tension in the fascia; but this really is a last resort and given that most cases will get better in time, I think an operation should be avoided if at all possible.

DR DAWN'S HEALTH CHECK
How to avoid cramp

Cramp is a common problem, and one in three people over the age of 60 often suffers with it. Although we don't know exactly what causes cramp, we do know there are several things that make us more prone to it. Here are my top tips for reducing your risk:

- Drink plenty of water.
- Avoid overexercising – tired muscles are more prone to cramp.
- Stretch your muscles before going to bed.
- Cut down your alcohol intake.
- Ask your doctor if any of your medications could be making things worse – water tablets (diuretics), some blood pressure and asthma medicines, and mental health drugs can all exacerbate cramp, but don't stop any medication without your doctor's advice.
- Try quinine tablets – taken at night they can relieve the symptoms.

VERRUCAS

These are wart-like growths found on the soles of the feet most commonly, but not always, in children. They are caused by a virus called the human papillomavirus, of which there are around 100 types. Personally, if a verruca is not causing pain, I suggest that parents leave it alone because verrucas will eventually clear up without treatment, and as long as the child covers his or her feet (particularly around swimming pools) to prevent spreading the virus, they won't come to any harm.

IS IT A VERRUCA OR A CORN?

If you are not sure whether it is a verruca or a corn, try paring it down with a pumice stone. If it's a verruca you will see lots of tiny spots, which are actually minute blood vessels, while a corn won't change its appearance.

WHAT YOU CAN DO

There are many over-the-counter remedies available for treating verrucas; ask your pharmacist for advice. If you are trying such a remedy, first soak the verruca in warm water for five minutes and remove any dead tissue with a pumice stone or emery board. When you apply the lotion make sure the whole verruca is painted and then cover with a plaster. You will have to be patient – the process needs to be repeated every day and may take several weeks to work. If this doesn't work and the verruca is troublesome, see your doctor. He or she may suggest

treatment by freezing the verruca. This is effective in about 75 per cent of cases but it can be quite painful and may need to be repeated several times.

You can reduce the risk of passing on verrucas (or picking them up in the first place) by not walking barefoot in communal changing areas at swimming pools – wear flip-flops or get verruca socks from your chemist.

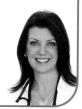

> **DR DAWN'S HEALTH CHECK**
> ### How do I treat a corn?
> Corns are a build-up of hard skin as a result of pressure. Here are some tips for dealing with them:
> - Wear well-fitting shoes that don't rub.
> - Try soaking your feet then rubbing down the corn with a pumice stone.
> - Corn plasters can help to break down the hard skin but should not be used by people with diabetes.

SWOLLEN ANKLES

This condition is common in pregnancy and is also generally more common in women than men. Apart from pregnancy, swollen ankles can be a sign of an underlying heart, kidney, or liver problem, and you should have a check-up with your doctor to rule these out. If the swelling is caused by an accumulation of fluid, your doctor may prescribe pills to prevent water retention (diuretics).

PREVENTING SWOLLEN ANKLES

There are also several things you can do to help yourself. Long periods of inactivity, during a long-haul flight, for example, hot weather, and pregnancy are common causes of swollen ankles, and with the these simple measures should make things significantly better:
- Don't stand still for long periods of time. If you have to stand, shifting from foot to foot will keep your calf muscles contracting and help pump blood back up to the heart, preventing the build-up of fluid in your ankles.
- If you are on a long-haul flight, try to get up and walk

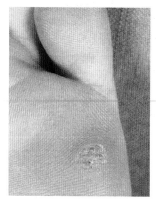

◄ *Verrucas can be identified by the presence of tiny spots in them.*

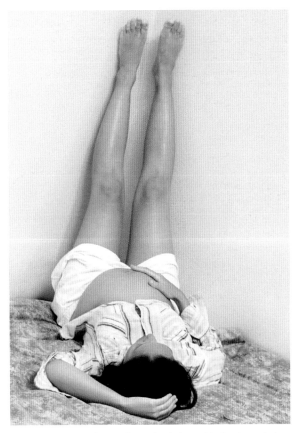

▲ Laying down with your feet raised above hip level can help alleviate swollen ankles, during pregnancy, for example.

around at regular intervals during the flight and take a brisk walk when you reach your destination.

- If you have to sit, try to keep your legs up and avoid sitting cross-legged.
- Wear support tights or the type of socks sold to help prevent deep vein thrombosis.
- Try taking a extract of red vine leaves, which helps maintain healthy leg veins and capillaries. You will need to take it every day for at least six weeks before you will notice any improvement, but persevere – it has helped many of my patients.

FLAT FEET

The human foot is designed to arch from front to back and from side to side. Almost all children start life with flat feet. They don't develop the normal arches until they have been walking for a while – usually between the ages of three and ten. Parents often worry about flat feet, but they are rarely a cause for concern.

FLAT FEET IN CHILDREN

There are a couple of simple tests you can do to check that your child's feet are normal:

- With your child standing upright, raise the big toe – the arch of the foot should become noticeable.
- Ask your child to stand on tiptoes – again, the arch should become prominent.

If the arches can be produced in this way, there is almost certainly nothing to worry about, and other than buying shoes with good arch supports, your child is unlikely to need any further treatment.

FLAT FEET IN ADULTS

Flat feet in adults often run in families and may be the result of degenerative changes in the joints in the middle of the foot, or because of tendon problems. Flat feet occur most commonly in women aged over 40 who lead fairly sedentary lives. In men, they are more likely to occur as a result of injury.

SHOULD I WORRY IF I HAVE FLAT FEET?

Probably not – most people with flat feet have no problems at all. You only need to see a doctor, chiropodist, or a podiatrist if you:

- Have pain in your feet despite well-fitting shoes.
- Wear out your shoes very quickly.
- Think your feet are getting stiff or flatter.
- Notice abnormal sensation or weakness in your feet.

FIND OUT MORE
www.bofss.org.uk

A woman produces, on average, 500 mature eggs during her fertile lifetime • Human eggs are the largest human cell, weighing as much as 175,000 sperm cells • Women lose up to 400 litres (700 pints) of blood during menstruation in a lifetime • Before puberty, girls have about half a million follicles containing immature eggs in their ovaries • Women who have hysterectomies are likely to have an earlier menopause • In a female fetus the uterus, fallopian tubes, and vagina start to develop by the 12th week of pregnancy

13

Women's health

Introduction It could be argued that what makes a woman is two breasts, a uterus (womb) and two ovaries. Women's health of course covers all aspects of medicine but in this chapter, I will concentrate on the health concerns involving these parts of our bodies.

The change from girl to woman can begin as early as nine with the development of breast buds (small swellings under the nipple). This may be very slow and asymmetrical to start with, but about a year after the breasts become noticeable, girls grow fine pubic hair which becomes darker and curlier over time.

Periods can begin any time from age 11 to 15. The exact timing is slightly dependent on body weight – they are unlikely to start before a girl weighs 47kg (104lb). A period is the shedding of the womb lining, noticed as vaginal bleeding, in response to hormones, and although they may be erratic at first they should settle into a regular cycle within two years. The exact length of our menstrual cycle depends on how long it takes for our eggs to develop. If an egg is not fertilized we will have a period 14 days after we ovulate. In a 28-day cycle that is also 14 days after our last period, but some women have longer cycles because their eggs take longer to mature.

PERIODS

The average age for girls to start their periods in this country is 12, and on average women in the UK are aged 50–52 when they go through the menopause and their periods stop. A menstrual cycle is typically 28 days long, but anything from 22 to 35 is regarded as normal. A period will normally last for five to seven days, and your blood loss can be anything up to 80ml (3fl oz). However, few women stroll through life with totally "normal" periods, and one in 20 will see their doctor every year with period problems.

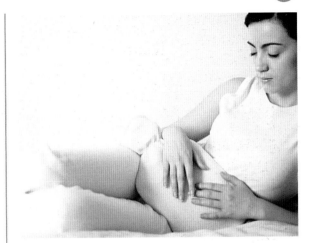

▲ Placing a heat pad on your tummy can help to ease painful periods.

WHAT CAUSES PAINFUL PERIODS?

Painful periods (or dysmenorrhoea) are common and affect most women at some point. Periods tend to become painful six months to a year after they first start. Painful periods are more common in young women, but they often settle spontaneously when you are in your thirties or after you have children, whichever comes first. It also runs in families (so if your mother or sister had problems, you are more likely to). Painful periods are also more common in smokers. Occasionally, painful periods are the result of a condition called endometriosis (see p.145).

You will have lighter, less painful periods if you are taking the contraceptive pill, so it can be a useful treatment if you also need contraception. Your doctor can also prescribe anti-inflammatory medication that is specifically aimed at relieving period pain. However, if you don't want to go down that route there are lots of other options open to you, see health check box, left.

SPOTTING BETWEEN PERIODS

If you do experience spotting between periods, you should see your doctor. Spotting between periods could indicate the presence of chlamydia (see p.169), and it's essential that you get it checked out. It may simply be that you have missed your contraceptive pill, or it can be stress-related, but it is always a good idea to have a swab test to check.

BLEEDING AFTER INTERCOURSE

It's important to see your doctor if you bleed after sex. It could be caused by an infection, but the most common reason I see for this is an ectropion (or erosion) on the cervix. It's not sinister, but can cause bleeding after intercourse. It is a condition that is easily treated – a special paint is applied to the cervix and it can be done as an outpatient procedure.

DR DAWN'S HEALTH CHECK
Easing painful periods
Here are my tips for relieving painful periods:
• Take pain-relief tablets such as paracetamol or aspirin.
• Put a heat pad on your lower tummy and/or your lower back.
• Avoid stress if you can, or try to reduce it.
• Take regular exercise.
• Take vitamin supplements – some women find vitamins B1, B12, and E helpful.
• The herbal remedy toki-shakuyaku-san can help.
• Acupuncture helps some women.
• TENS machines also help. They work by creating high-frequency nerve stimulation that causes a tingling sensation on your skin, distracting your brain from focusing on the period pain.

WHEN SHOULD YOU WORRY ABOUT ABSENT PERIODS?

Any sexually active woman of childbearing age who misses a period should do a pregnancy test – no form of contraception is 100 per cent guaranteed. If you exercise excessively or you are underweight (a BMI of less than 18.5, see p.94), this can stop your periods too. Simply cutting back on the exercise or gaining some weight may be all that you need to do. If your periods stop for more than six months, you should see your doctor for some blood tests to check your hormone levels.

HEAVY PERIODS

One in three women has greater than average blood loss (referred to as heavy periods or menorrhagia) and, unlike painful periods, this often becomes more frequent with age. It accounts for many of the 45,000 hysterectomies performed in this country every year. But a hysterectomy is a major operation, taking anything up to 12 weeks to recover from, and shouldn't be undertaken lightly, particularly as there are now several other treatments available. Occasionally, heavy periods are the result of a condition called endometriosis (see p.145).

• The contraceptive pill can help. As long as you are slim, don't smoke, and have no other risk factors (see p.167), it's safe to take the pill until your menopause.

• There are two anti-inflammatory treatments available on prescription that are specifically licensed to help reduce the flow of heavy periods.

• Have an IUS coil fitted. This is a small contraceptive device that secretes tiny amounts of progestogen hormone (about the same as taking two minipills a week), which prevents the lining of the uterus from thickening. It lasts for five years and many women find their periods stop altogether or certainly become significantly lighter. This can be fitted at the family planning clinic.

• Your doctor may refer you for an endometrial ablation. This is a minor operation in which the lining of the uterus is removed. You will need a general anaesthetic, but you're normally only in for the day, and you will back to normal within a fortnight. The procedure is successful for nine out of ten women.

PREMENSTRUAL SYNDROME

Often referred to as PMS, this affects about one and a half million women in this country. Over a hundred different symptoms have been attributed to it, but irritability and bloating are the two that seem to cause the most distress. Although as many as three out of four women suffer mild symptoms at some point, premenstrual syndrome often gets worse in your thirties and forties.

WHAT YOU CAN DO

The first thing I ask my patients to do is to keep a symptom diary – true PMS develops in the week or two leading up to a period, then subsides within a couple of days of your period starting.

TREATMENT

Finding a treatment for premenstrual syndrome is like choosing a dress – one size doesn't fit all. The only things that have been consistently shown to work are water tablets, anti-inflammatory medication, and some antidepressants. However, there are lots of alternatives

▼ St John's wort may help to reduce the symptoms of PMS.

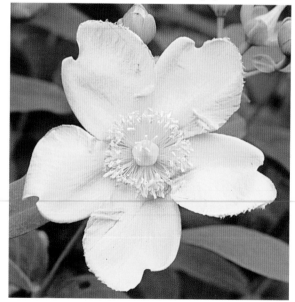

that have helped some of my patients and may be worth a try.

• Try taking Agnus castus extract or St John's wort (although St John's wort may reduce the effectiveness of oral contraceptives, so don't take it before consulting your doctor if you are on the pill).

• Talk to your doctor about one of the new generation contraceptive pills. Taking the pills continuously (missing the pill-free weeks) eases some women's symptoms.

• Increase your exercise levels.

• Try cognitive behavioural therapy.

• In extreme cases, doctors can medically "switch off" your ovaries, or they can be removed with an operation.

FIND OUT MORE
www.pms.org.uk

FIBROIDS

These are benign tumours that develop in the uterus. They are extremely common. About half of all 50-year-old women have them, and most cause no symptoms at all. Fibroids tend to run in families and are oestrogen-dependent, so shrink after your menopause (unless you take HRT).

TREATMENT

About one-quarter of the women with fibroids develop problems, mainly heavy bleeding. Until recently, many of these women ended up having a hysterectomy, but a new treatment, which involves removing only the lining of the uterus (an endometrial ablation) has meant a dramatic reduction in the number of hysterectomies performed each year.

I am often asked if fibroids could become cancerous. The answer is that in theory they can, but the chance is about one in a million and I have never seen it happen.

PREGNANCY

Pregnancy is a huge time of change for any woman, and it is normal to experience a variety of complaints during the time from conception to delivery. Pregnancy is a huge subject to which entire books are devoted, so although I won't go into great detail here, there are a few essential points that I would like to cover.

PREGNANCY TESTS

You can ask your doctor for a pregnancy test or you can do it yourself at home. Over-the-counter pregnancy test kits are extremely reliable – so much so that if a woman comes into my surgery with a positive test, I don't generally repeat it. (One exception to this would be for a woman who felt pregnant but had a negative test.)

DR DAWN'S HEALTH CHECK
Before trying for a baby

If you are thinking of starting (or extending) your family, now is a good time to:

• Make sure you are up to date with your smear tests.

• Ask your doctor to check whether you are immune to rubella. This involves a blood test but is well worth doing. Rubella infection during pregnancy can cause blindness, deafness, and mental development problems in your baby. If your blood test shows you are not immune, your doctor will be able to offer you a vaccination.

• Start taking folic acid – 4mg per day. Research has shown that this dose taken for three months before conception and for the first three months of your pregnancy reduces the risk of spina bifida affecting the baby.

• If you smoke, give up now (see p.70)

• Keep your alcohol intake to recommended limits.

• Maintain a healthy weight. Not only will this help you to conceive, it will also mean you're less likely to have any complications in pregnancy.

• If you are taking any prescription medicines, talk to your doctor as you may need to change them. Whatever you do, don't stop any medicines without talking to your doctor first.

WHAT ARE THE SYMPTOMS?

The symptoms of early pregnancy, aside from the obviously missed period, include:

• Nausea – note that I don't call it "morning sickness". Feeling sick can start even before your first period is missed and it doesn't necessarily restrict itself to mornings. Eight out of ten women in their first pregnancy suffer some nausea, but the good news is that it usually starts to improve by 12 weeks and disappears by 16 weeks.

• Swollen or tender breasts.

• Needing to wee more often (urinary frequency), which tends to start around six weeks.

• Extreme tiredness.

WHAT YOU CAN DO IF YOU ARE PREGNANT

Assuming this is a happy event, you need to tell your doctor's surgery as soon as possible. Some practices will want you to see your doctor; others will book you in to see a midwife. While you are waiting for your appointment, you should concentrate on giving your unborn baby the best start in life, so:

• If you are still a smoker, give up now.

• Make sure you are eating a well-balanced diet. However, don't eat peanuts, raw eggs, liver, soft cheese, or pâté, all of which can be harmful.

• Ideally, cut out alcohol; at the very least limit it to one or two units once or twice a week (see p.77 for the amount of alcohol that constitutes one unit).

• Keep exercising sensibly – now is not the time to take up a challenging new training programme, but regular exercise will be good for you and your growing baby.

• Start taking folic acid, 4mg per day (if you are not already doing so).

• Rest when you need it; you may find it difficult not to.

It is normal to experience different feelings and symptoms during pregnancy, but if you are worried about something specific then don't be afraid to seek medical advice.

? **DID YOU KNOW**

If you have had unprotected sex and don't want to be pregnant?

You can take the so-called "morning after pill". This name is actually a misnomer, as it can be taken any time up to 72 hours after unprotected sex, although the sooner you take it the better. It is available over the counter from your chemist so there is no need to wait for your doctor's surgery to open on Monday morning. If you have gone beyond the 72-hour window, call your doctor or family planning clinic as a coil can be fitted up to five days after you had sex.

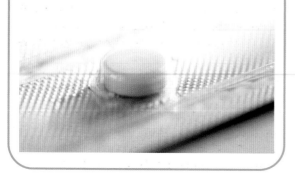

DR DAWN'S HEALTH CHECK
Coping with miscarriage

At least one in five pregnancies ends in miscarriage. Most early miscarriages are probably due to a chromosome abnormality – a one-off mistake in the transfer of genetic material, meaning it is unlikely to happen again.

Miscarriage is an extremely distressing experience for a woman and her partner, but it may help a little to remember the following:

• Although it is difficult, try to remain positive. You will have a much greater chance of having a successful pregnancy than of having another miscarriage the next time around.

• Take the time and the space that you need to deal with your emotions. Women who miscarry have the tendency to feel guilty, but remember that miscarriage is rarely anything to do with something you have or haven't done, so don't blame yourself.

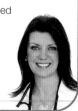

FIND OUT MORE
www.ukpregnancy.com

CERVICAL SMEARS

Smear tests look for changes in your cervix, which if left untreated could progress to cancer over a period of years. So having a regular smear test can prevent you from developing the cancer. It may not be your idea of a fun day out but it's really worth having it done regularly. It's estimated that cervical screening saves around 4,500 lives in England every year.

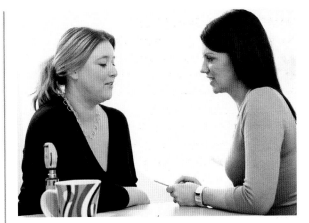

▲ Your doctor will be able to talk you through any concerns you have relating to smear test results.

HOW OFTEN SHOULD I HAVE A SMEAR?

All women registered with a National Health Service doctor will be invited to attend the surgery for a smear test when they reach the age of 25. Provided everything is normal, you will be invited back every three years until you are 49. After 50 you will be invited every five years and, as long as your results stay normal, you will stop being called for smear tests after you are 65.

The start point has changed: previously girls were recommended to have their first smear at the age of 21 and I am often asked if delaying it until 25 is safe. In fact, the decision was made on good grounds. Cervical cancer under the age of 25 is thankfully exceptionally rare and women's bodies and cervixes are still developing and changing in their early twenties. The changes noted on smears in the younger age group were often reported as abnormal, necessitating follow-up smears. These changes settle, but being recalled for smear tests causes understandable angst, so it was decided to change the starting age for the screening programme.

WHAT HAPPENS DURING A SMEAR TEST?

When you attend your smear test appointment, you will be asked about your periods and any hormones or other medication you may be taking. You will then be asked to undress from the waist down and lie on your back on an examination couch. (If you are wearing a full skirt you should be able to hitch it up – there is no need to remove it completely.) The nurse or doctor will then ask you to bend your knees, and relax your legs open. She will insert a small instrument called a speculum into your vagina so that she can see the cervix. Using a wooden spatula or plastic brush, she will wipe the cervix to collect some cells. These cells are then sent to the laboratory for analysis. The whole process will take around 10 minutes and isn't painful.

CAN I ASK FOR MY SMEAR TO BE DONE BY A WOMAN?

Yes, you can – just ask at the time of booking. In many practices cervical smear tests are done by the practice nurse and they often tend to be women, but if you are concerned then just ask.

CAN I HAVE A SMEAR DURING MY PERIOD?

No – a smear cannot be taken during your period because blood obscures the view of the cells down a microscope, so it's worth remembering this when making your appointment.

CAN I HAVE SEX BEFORE A SMEAR?

Yes, you can. However, if you use a spermicide, a barrier method of contraception, or any lubricant during sex, then you should abstain for 24 hours before your smear test as the chemicals may make it difficult to interpret the test.

IF I AM PREGNANT, WILL MY DOCTOR DO A SMEAR TEST?

It is very unlikely for two reasons. The hormonal changes that occur in pregnancy can cause cervical changes that could affect the result of the test. In addition, whenever possible, doctors wouldn't choose to initiate any treatment until after a baby is born. So unless it is absolutely necessary, doctors avoid taking a smear during pregnancy.

I HAVE HAD A HYSTERECTOMY – DO I STILL NEED A SMEAR TEST?

This will depend on why you had the hysterectomy and what type of hysterectomy you had. Occasionally, a subtotal hysterectomy is performed, in which the cervix is left in place, in which case you need a smear test. If your hysterectomy was done for cervical cancer, you will need to attend for what we call vault smears – check with your doctor.

I HAVE HAD AN ABNORMAL SMEAR – WHY DO I HAVE TO WAIT SIX MONTHS FOR A REPEAT TEST?

Minor cervical changes usually improve over a period of about six months without the need for any treatment, which is why we leave it. If your follow-up smear is normal, you may be called back six to 12 months later to check that the cervix is still fine, then you'll go back to a normal three-year recall. If, however, your follow-up smear test shows changes, you will probably be referred for a special test called a colposcopy in which the cervix can be examined more closely and abnormal cells can be removed.

WHAT IS AN "INADEQUATE" RESULT?

Around one in ten smear tests are reported as "inadequate". This usually means that either there weren't enough cells to give a normal result, or the cells couldn't be properly assessed because the view was obscured by blood or mucus. In this instance, your doctor will ask you to come back for another smear in three months, when the cells have recovered enough to repeat the test.

DO LESBIANS NEED SMEAR TESTS?

The risks of purely gay sex are not known but are likely to be very small indeed. However, many lesbian women have had heterosexual relationships in the past, in which case they should definitely attend for regular smear tests.

CERVICAL CANCER

Cervical cancer usually develops slowly over several years, which is why regular cervical screening is essential to detect changes early and prevent it occurring. However, around 3,000 women are still diagnosed with cervical cancer every year in the UK.

TYPES OF CERVICAL CANCER

There are two types of cervical cancer:
- Squamous cell carcinoma – this is by far the commonest form and is due to cancerous changes in the flat cells that cover the outer surface of the cervix.
- Adenocarcinoma – a rarer form of cancer that starts in the glandular cells lining the inside of the neck of the uterus. It can be more difficult to detect with smear tests.

WHAT ARE THE SYMPTOMS?

Most women with cervical cancer will not have any symptoms until the disease is quite advanced – this is another reason why it is so important to attend for your smears when you are called. Cervical cancer can cause abnormal bleeding so if you have any bleeding between your periods, you should see your doctor to rule out this possibility. However, most cancers of the cervix are picked up on routine smear tests before any symptoms are present.

WHAT IS THE TREATMENT?

Treatment depends on how early the disease is diagnosed, and can involve any combination of radiotherapy, chemotherapy, and surgery. Early stage cervical cancer has an excellent outlook, with 85 per cent of women making a full recovery, but sadly more advanced disease that has spread beyond the cervix doesn't have such a good outlook – around 1,000 British women still die of the disease each year.

FIND OUT MORE
www.cervicalcancer.uk.com

POLYCYSTIC OVARY SYNDROME

Sometimes abbreviated to PCOS, this is one of the most common hormonal problems to affect women. Some experts believe as many as one in five women has the condition. It is caused by an increase in your ovarian androgen production and leads to an accumulation of underdeveloped follicles in your ovaries.

WHAT ARE THE SYMPTOMS?

Classic symptoms include:
- Weight gain.
- Unwanted facial hair.
- Irregular periods.
- Acne.

Women with this condition genuinely find it difficult to lose weight, which seems doubly cruel given that, for many, weight loss actually improves all the other symptoms.

Polycystic ovary syndrome affects women differently, so not everyone will have weight problems, for example. For some women the symptoms will be mild, but sadly for others they are more marked. The diagnosis is made using ultrasound and blood tests.

CAN IT BE TREATED?

The hormonal imbalance of polycystic ovary syndrome can be treated with the contraceptive pill and a drug used in diabetes called metformin. Women with PCOS are often referred to as subfertile and need to take a drug called clomifene to help them ovulate if they are trying to conceive. The ovaries can also be stimulated with keyhole surgery using a technique called diathermy.

As tough as it may be, weight loss is worth working at – it will improve skin, hair and fertility.

FIND OUT MORE
www.verity-pcos.org.uk

ENDOMETRIOSIS

This is a condition in which deposits of uterine tissue are found outside your uterus, attached to other organs in the abdomen. The tissue is just as sensitive to hormones as your uterine lining, so it is shed during the course of your menstrual cycle, and can cause abdominal pain.

WHAT ARE THE SYMPTOMS?

Endometriosis does not always cause symptoms, but if they do occur they are likely to include:
- Pain in the lower abdomen.
- Heavy periods.
- Pain during sexual intercourse.

Women with endometriosis often find it difficult to conceive and, in fact, a diagnosis is frequently only made during investigation for subfertility.

HOW IS IT DIAGNOSED?

I think endometriosis is one of the most underdiagnosed conditions. It's not uncommon for women to suffer for many years before finally being diagnosed with endometriosis. It can't be seen on a blood test or a scan. The only way to make the diagnosis is to look in the pelvis with a special telescope called a laparoscope.

CAN IT BE TREATED?

The only proven treatments are either hormones (which reduce your fertility) or surgical removal of the deposits. The latter can be technically difficult, depending on where the deposits are, and time-consuming, but often results in improved fertility.

Lots of my patients have tried complementary therapies to help the pain, including acupuncture, relaxation techniques, and aromatherapy. None of these will cure it, but they have helped some individuals so may be worth a try.

FIND OUT MORE
www.endo.org.uk

THRUSH

This is a condition caused by a yeast called *Candida albicans* that lives harmlessly in your gut and on your skin. One in five women has this fungus inside their vagina without any sign of infection but sometimes it proliferates, causing the classic symptoms of burning, itching, and a creamy discharge.

WHO DOES IT AFFECT?

Most women have an attack of thrush at some time in their lives. It is common in pregnancy, and women with diabetes are far more susceptible to thrush because of their high blood-sugar levels. Conversely, if you suffer from recurrent attacks you should ask your doctor to check you for diabetes.

WHAT YOU CAN DO

Thrush is not technically a sexually transmitted infection, although it can be passed between partners during intercourse. The first time you have an attack of thrush, go to your doctor so that he or she can confirm the diagnosis. Subsequent attacks can be treated with creams and pessaries readily available from a chemist.

DR DAWN'S HEALTH CHECK
Keeping thrush at bay

- Avoid tight jeans.
- Wear underwear that is cotton only.
- Avoid antibiotics unless absolutely necessary – they kill off the good bugs that live in the vagina and keep thrush under control.
- Avoid perfumed soaps and bubble baths that alter the pH of your skin, making it easier for the yeast to multiply. Some women also find a few drops of tea-tree oil in the bath helps.
- Keep stress to a minimum.
- Eat a balanced diet to boost the immune system.
- Change your tampons regularly.
- Always wipe from front to back after going to the loo.
- Try eating probiotic yoghurt. Some of my patients also use it directly in the vagina and find it very soothing.

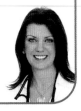

VAGINAL DISCHARGE

Every week I see women in my surgery who are concerned about their vaginal discharge. In fact, as many as one in ten women will see their doctor every year complaining of a discharge. Often the discharge is completely normal but sometimes it can result from an infection or another problem.

HOW DO YOU KNOW IF THE DISCHARGE IS NORMAL?

The lining of your vagina is like the inside of your mouth. It produces secretions that help to keep it healthy. Normal secretions tend to be clear or milky and odourless and shouldn't be accompanied by other symptoms. The secretions change during your menstrual cycle; they are generally more pronounced in the middle of the month around the time of ovulation, when they tend to thicken and look more like egg white. They can also change if you are stressed, when you are sexually aroused, pregnant, and even if you take the contraceptive pill.

The normal pH of your vagina is slightly acidic – it's kept this way by healthy bacteria living there. Women who notice a change in their vaginal secretions often take frequent baths, using a lot of soap, thinking they will improve the problem. In fact, this can make it worse as perfumed soaps can alter the pH, making the vagina more prone to infection. Douching with water from the shower head is all that you need to do to freshen up.

WHEN TO SEEK MEDICAL ADVICE

If you notice that your discharge is a different colour or smell or you also have burning or itching sensation, then it's worth getting it checked by your doctor. A simple swab test may be all that is necessary to check things out. The most common explanation is an infection, but sometimes it's caused by a forgotten tampon or an erosion or raw area on your cervix, all of which can be easily treated.

If your doctor doesn't find anything wrong but you are still unhappy with the amount of discharge, it may be worth changing to a progestogen-dominant contraceptive as these tend to dry the vagina.

MENOPAUSE

On average, women in this country experience the menopause between the ages of 50 and 52, although it tends to be earlier in women who smoke. Women tend to follow a similar pattern to their mothers, so ask yours if you can.

WHAT ARE THE SIGNS AND SYMPTOMS?

Menopausal symptoms can include anything from dry skin and joint pain, to tiredness and memory problems, but the classic symptoms are hot flushes, night sweats, and mood swings. Around 70 per cent of women experience them. Why the remaining 30 per cent experience the same hormonal changes without the symptoms is not clear, but having seen how difficult the menopause can be for many women, I would like to be one of latter group when my time comes!

WHAT'S THE STORY ON HRT NOW?

HRT has helped many women and five or ten years ago, I would pretty much have advocated putting HRT in the water. However, some large studies into the potential risks of HRT have changed all that and scary headlines have put hundreds of women off even considering it. I would like to take the opportunity to put things into perspective here. There is no doubt that taking HRT is associated with an increased risk of heart disease, stroke, and breast cancer. But the risks are small, and HRT is by no means all bad. It actually protects against osteoporosis (see p.116) and colon cancer.

WHAT EXACTLY ARE THE RISKS OF HRT?

So let's take a look at the figures. In a group of 10,000 women aged 50 or over who do not take HRT, you can expect that each year 30 would develop heart disease, 30 would be diagnosed with breast cancer, and 21 would have a stroke. If that same group of women were on combined HRT, there would be an extra seven cases of heart disease, an additional eight breast cancers, and eight more strokes. But there is also another way to look at it: having a BMI over 30 (see p.94) increases your risk of breast cancer by more than taking HRT. Now, if your mother has had a heart attack or your sister has breast

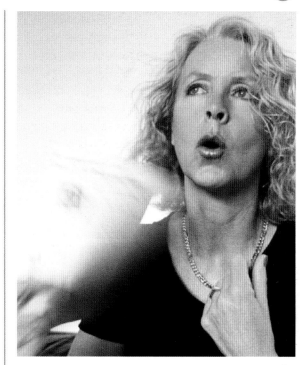

▲ *The menopause can make you extremely sensitive to heat changes, causing hot flushes.*

cancer, then even those small increased risks may be too much for you to consider HRT. But for the many women who struggle with menopausal symptoms, a short course may be all they need to get back on track.

WHY DOES HRT SEEM TO BE SAFER IN YOUNGER WOMEN?

The risks aren't the same if you have an early menopause. This is partly because younger women have lower risks of heart disease and breast cancer anyway, but also because the risk associated with oestrogen is cumulative. Women who experience an early menopause and choose to take HRT are only replacing what they would naturally be expected to have had until they are 50. The clock only starts ticking in terms of HRT risk after the age of 50.

IS HRT RIGHT FOR ME?

Don't automatically rule it out. If you are struggling with hot flushes or a total loss of self-confidence, talk to your doctor. Life is not black and white; your doctor can assess your individual risks against the benefits of HRT so that you can make an informed choice.

OTHER CONCERNS ABOUT THE MENOPAUSE

Every woman's experience of the menopause is different. Below are some of the questions I am most frequently asked in surgery.

How can I deal with vaginal dryness?

A lot of women notice that the natural secretions in their vagina dry up as they go through the menopause. This can make sex uncomfortable and often causes symptoms of cystitis (see p.107). Dryness can be easily treated by putting oestrogen in the form of a pessary or cream into your vagina. The hormone works locally and only a minimal amount is absorbed, so it doesn't carry the risks of conventional HRT but can revolutionize your life. If you don't want to take hormones at all, you can try a slow-release lubricant like Replens (available from your chemist). Place it in your vagina and replace it every few days.

What causes the hot flushes?

It is thought that during the menopause the part of our brain that's responsible for temperature control becomes oversensitive. Your body experiences tiny changes in temperature throughout the day and normally you are totally unaware of them. You only sweat when the temperature changes are major, for example when you have a fever. Menopausal women can be so sensitive

▼ Caffeine can make hot flushes worse, so cutting it out of your diet may help.

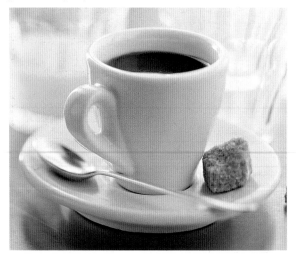

to temperature changes that they flush with every tiny temperature fluctuation – sometimes even when drinking a warm drink.

Alcohol, caffeine, and monosodium glutamate (food flavour enhancer) can make things even worse so try to cut these out of your diet.

How long will I have menopausal flushes?

That's a bit like asking how long is a piece of string! Flushes last on average about two years, but I have met some women who are still having them after 15 years.

Do you get menopause symptoms after stopping HRT?

You may find that when you stop HRT you have some menopausal symptoms, but in my experience they are usually less severe and shorter-lived. When you go through a natural menopause, your hormones are in turmoil. They don't just fade away quietly and it's this variation in hormone levels that seems to cause the symptoms. By weaning patients off HRT gradually, I often find I can keep their symptoms to a minimum. There are lots of tricks that can be used, such as taking HRT on alternate days or cutting patches in half, but your doctor will be able to advise you.

Can herbal treatments help?

I have seen a huge rise in the interest in herbal treatments for menopausal symptoms in recent years, and it may be worth experimenting with different things:
• Black cohosh seems to relieve the sweats and flushes for a lot of women. Take 8mg of standardized extract daily, and be prepared to persevere for three months as it doesn't work overnight.
• Vitamin E and evening primrose oil supplements may also help with flushes.
• Other popular remedies include red clover and soy protein.
• Agnus castus is also worth a try if it's mood swings that are your biggest concern. Vitamin B6 supplement (10mg daily) has helped some of my patients.

The important thing to remember when taking any herbal supplements is that you should stop using them if you experience any side effects, and if you are taking any other form of medication then you should check with your doctor first. It is also extremely important to maintain a healthy diet during the menopause, so make sure you are getting enough vitamins and minerals in your daily diet.

Are there any non-hormonal drug treatments?

Yes. An old-fashioned blood pressure drug called clonidine works well at stopping hot flushes and I use it for women who have too high a risk of breast cancer to consider taking HRT. Some antidepressants may help the hot flushes and mood problems associated with the menopause.

> **FIND OUT MORE**
> www.amarantmenopausetrust.org.uk

PAINFUL BREASTS (MASTALGIA)

Seven out of ten women experience breast pain at some time or other. This is often linked to poorly fitting bras, so a proper bra fitter should be your first port of call. Underwired bras can make the problem worse and you must wear a well-fitting sports bra during exercise.

WHAT YOU CAN DO

Reducing caffeine intake and the amount of fat in your diet can also help with painful breasts. Try taking evening primrose oil if the breast pain seems to be related to your periods. The active ingredient in evening primrose oil is a substance called gammalinolenic acid (GLA) and if you are going to take it you will need 240mg of GLA a day for at least three months. I often see women who have tried evening primrose oil and say it didn't work for them, but when we talk in more detail I find they have usually taken a lower dose or haven't taken it for long enough. Evening primrose oil doesn't work for everyone, but it's worth giving it a try.

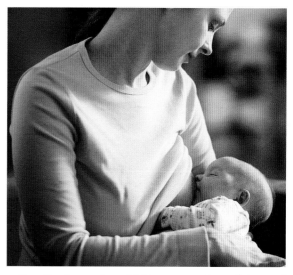

▲ *Breastfeeding can be painful for some mothers.*

Getting the right fitting bra is extremely important, but bear in mind that your breasts may change size over the course of your menstrual cycle. If you do notice that your bra is particularly uncomfortable because your breasts are larger before your period, it may be worth investing in a larger bra size for these times. If all this fails, then talk to your doctor about possible prescription drugs.

> **DR DAWN'S HEALTH CHECK**
> **Pregnancy and breastfeeding**
>
> Pregnancy is a common trigger of breast pain, as even in the early stages of pregnancy your body will be preparing to breastfeed your baby. For your breasts, that means an increased blood supply and an increase in size as they accumulate fat and the milk glands mature, which can mean a change of one or two cup sizes. For most women, the symptoms settle by week 14 and, although the breasts remain bigger, the tenderness goes.
>
> Breastfeeding can also cause pain for some mothers. If you have painful swollen breasts, your milk may not be flowing effectively. Get help to check the position of your baby while he or she is feeding, as a poor position may stop the baby from emptying the breast. If you have continuing problems with pain during breastfeeding, speak to your doctor or health visitor.

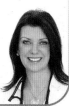

BREAST LUMPS

Any woman discovering a new breast lump automatically thinks the worst. In fact, nine out of ten lumps seen by breast specialists are not malignant. So what are these lumps and how do we tell the difference? The most common breast lumps are fibroadenomas and breast cysts.

FIBROADENOMAS

As a general rule, these lumps, also called "breast mice" because they can be moved about under the skin, tend to occur in women aged between 15 and 30. The younger you are when you develop them, the more likely they are to disappear spontaneously.

BREAST CYSTS

Cysts (fluid-filled sacs) are more common in women aged between 40 and 50. They are often multiple and why they occur is unclear. People have speculated that

▾ Becoming familiar with what your breasts look and feel like is an important part of being "breast aware".

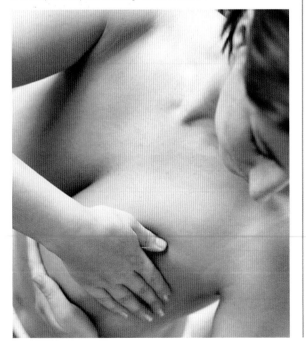

there may be a slight increased risk of breast cancer but if this is the case, it is likely to be very small indeed.

IF YOU NEED A BIOPSY

To the trained clinician, these lumps can feel different but, to be honest, the only way to be certain is to have a look at some cells or fluid under a microscope. This means inserting a needle into the lump and removing, or aspirating, the tissue. The results are usually available within a few days and the discomfort is a small price to pay for the reassurance that follows in most cases.

HOW OFTEN SHOULD I EXAMINE MY OWN BREASTS?

I don't like women to get too hung up on self-examination. The important thing is that every woman is "breast aware", and the following tips may help:

• Get to know what your breasts look and feel like – that way you are more likely to notice any changes in your breasts early on.

• Take time to look in the mirror. I often see women who have suddenly noticed that one breast is larger than the other or hangs down more. In fact, we are all asymmetrical and that is normal. It is a change in the appearance that can be significant.

• Use the flat of your hand to feel your breasts in a warm, soapy bath. Some women's breasts are lumpier than others, so get to know what is normal for you, and if you notice any change report it to your doctor straight away.

! SEEK MEDICAL ADVICE NOW
If you notice any of the following:

• A new lump.

• A bloody discharge from your nipple or any new discharge if you are over 50.

• Your nipple starts to invert. Nipples that have always been inverted are not a risk, but if your nipple starts to go in having always pointed outward, it could be a sign that there is a tumour underneath.

• The skin on your breast starts to dimple, looking like orange peel.

• Eczema around your nipple.

• A lump in your armpit.

BREAST CANCER

Breast cancer is the number one health concern for women and understandably so, given that it is the most common cancer of women in this country, killing around 15,000 women every year. In fact one in nine women in the UK develops breast cancer during their lifetime, but the earlier it's picked up, the better the outlook. Many women can expect to complete a normal lifespan with the disease provided they are treated early.

WHO GETS BREAST CANCER?

Anyone can develop breast cancer. About 41,000 women are diagnosed with the condition in the UK every year. Although it is rare, men can also get breast cancer. The main risk factors that make the disease more likely are listed in the box (right).

WHAT ABOUT THE BREAST CANCER GENE?

Experts believe that as many as one in ten breast cancers may be caused by a genetic predisposition due to an abnormal or mutated gene, and so far three such genes have been identified – BRCA1, BRCA2, and BRCA3. Interestingly, the BRCA genes are designed to protect against cancerous changes but small changes in their structure mean that they lose their protective effect, leaving the individual more prone to cancer of the breast as well as the bowel, ovary and, to a lesser extent, the uterus.

Any woman with a strong family history of these cancers may be eligible for genetic testing on the NHS and should discuss this with their doctor.

WHAT ABOUT HRT AND BREAST CANCER?

Hundreds of column inches have been written about the risks of breast cancer for women taking HRT. There is an increased risk, but things need to be put into perspective – if you took 1,000 women aged 65 who had never taken HRT, 50 of them would be expected to get breast cancer. If you took an identical group of women but had given them oestrogen-only HRT for five years, there would be one additional case of breast cancer. If that same group of women was given combined oestrogen

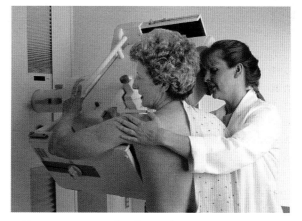

▲ *Mammograms are offered every three years to all women between the ages of 50 and 70.*

and progestogen HRT for five years, there would be six extra cases of breast cancer.

HRT does increase the risk of breast cancer and the longer you take it the greater the risk, but it is by no means all bad.

HOW IS BREAST CANCER DIAGNOSED?

Most breast cancers will first be detected when a woman notices a lump in her breast that is investigated further, and some are picked up during a routine mammography.

? DID YOU KNOW
Who is at risk?

The main risk factors include:

- Increasing age.
- Having one or more close relatives with the disease.
- Starting periods early (under 12).
- Having a late menopause (after 55).
- Having no children or having your first child after the age of 30.
- Being obese.
- Eating a high-fat diet.
- Drinking alcohol above recommended limits.
- Taking HRT.
- Exposure to radiation.

If I see a woman with a new lump just before her period, I usually arrange to see her again a week or two later after her period to check that it has gone. Any persistent lump should be referred to a specialist.

A breast specialist will examine both breasts, and will probably be able to make a good assessment of the lump's nature. However, as doctors can't always be 100 per cent certain, most women with a breast lump will be offered a mammogram. The specialist may also think it necessary to take a biopsy of the lump. This involves inserting a needle into the lump to remove cells or fluid for analysis under a microscope. The biopsy will be performed under local anaesthetic, so the procedure itself is uncomfortable rather than painful, and you may experience a little bruising afterwards.

WHAT IS A MAMMOGRAM?

A mammogram is a special X-ray of the breast. It involves placing each breast separately between two plates and then X-raying them. The process can feel quite uncomfortable but it doesn't take long – typically only a few minutes – and, in my opinion, the reassurance of a normal result that follows in the majority of cases is well worth the discomfort involved. Usually two X-ray pictures are taken – one from above and one from the side.

Mammography picks up around 90 per cent of breast cancers. That does mean that some cancers are missed, so even if a woman has a normal mammogram, she should continue to be breast aware and report any changes to her doctor.

MYTH BUSTERS
Let's take a look at some of the myths we hear about breast cancer.

ANTIPERSPIRANTS CAN CAUSE BREAST CANCER	FALSE	There has been an e-mail circulating for several years claiming that antiperspirant deodorants are a major cause of breast cancer. However, there is no evidence to support this. The theory is that they stop toxins being removed from the body and that these then build up in the lymphatic system, causing breast cancer. This is not true. First, sweat glands are completely different to lymph glands. Secondly, breast cancer starts in the breast and may spread to the lymph glands – it doesn't start in the lymphatic system.
		The theoretical link was based on the fact that scientists have found traces of substances called parabens (sometimes used in deodorants) in some breast tumours. Parabens do have some weak oestrogenic activity and we know that oestrogen is a factor in breast cancer, but the amounts found were tiny and 90 per cent of antiperspirants are now paraben-free.
WEARING AN UNDERWIRED BRA INCREASES YOUR RISK OF BREAST CANCER	FALSE	Again, the theory behind this myth is that the wire restricts the flow of toxins away from the breast, but there is absolutely no science to support this.
BREAST IMPLANTS INCREASE YOUR RISK OF BREAST CANCER	FALSE	There is no link between breast augmentation and breast cancer. However, having implants can make it more difficult for you to identify a new lump and make mammography more difficult to interpret so they could delay the diagnosis.

How often should I have a mammogram?

The NHS offers routine mammography to every woman between 50 and 70 every three years. Provided you are registered with an NHS doctor, you will automatically be called. Because the programme is constantly rolling, this may not necessarily be during your 50th year, but you will be called before your 53rd birthday.

Why are women under 50 not offered a mammogram?

Breast tissue is denser before the menopause, making it more difficult to interpret mammograms reliably, although technology is improving all the time. Breast cancer is also much less common pre-menopause. That said, women at high risk will be offered earlier screening.

Can I have a mammogram if I have implants?

Yes, but you should tell the radiographer that you have implants as they may need to adapt their technique to show as much breast tissue as possible.

HOW IS BREAST CANCER TREATED?

Treatment of breast cancer is variable and depends on a number of factors, including patient choice. The decisions on which treatments to use are based on:

- The size of the tumour.
- The grade of the tumour. Breast cancers are graded from 1–3, with grade 3 being the most aggressive.
- Whether the tumour has spread to the lymph nodes.
- Whether the tumour is sensitive to hormones.
- Whether the tumour has HER2 receptors.

Most women with breast cancer can expect to have a combination of:

- Surgery – this may involve removing a lump (lumpectomy) or all of the breast (mastectomy). Research has shown that lumpectomy and radiotherapy is as effective for most women as a mastectomy, and many women will end up with this option. However, for larger tumours a mastectomy may be the best option. It is normal for the patient to be involved in the decision-making process, but it can also be quite daunting. If you are struggling, a good question to ask your specialist is "What would you do if it was your relative?".
- Radiotherapy – this helps to prevent the cancer recurring. It may involve several visits to your local

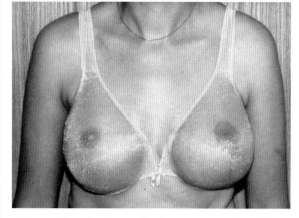

▲ *The good results of reconstructive surgery are shown here on the right breast following a mastectomy.*

radiotherapy centre and can leave you feeling extremely tired but it can be an effective treatment.

- Chemotherapy – not all breast cancers will require chemotherapy but if they do, it usually takes 4–6 months to complete the course. Side effects such as vomiting are common, but there are some excellent anti-sickness drugs available. Hair loss is another common problem.
- Hormonal therapies – women whose cancer cells have receptors for oestrogen are likely to be offered tamoxifen or a newer drug called an aromatase inhibitor, which they will probably need to take for five years.
- Trastuzumab (better known by its brand name, Herceptin) – some breast cancers have receptors on the cells called HER2 receptors and these cancers may respond to this drug, which is designed to attach to the receptors. It only works for about one in four breast cancers and is very expensive. Your specialist will be able to advise you as to whether your particular cancer would be suitable.

FIND OUT MORE
www.breastcancercare.org.uk

• Adult men are on average 13cm (5in) taller than women • All men have one testicle slightly lower than the other • Testicles will increase in size by 500 per cent during puberty • At their peak, adult testes produce over 100 million sperm every day • It takes 70 days to create a single sperm • A sperm is the smallest human cell.

14
Men's health

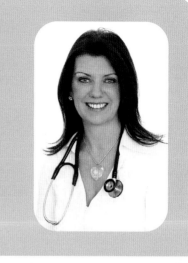

Introduction Men's health could cover just about any aspect of medicine but I will concentrate here on health issues involving the penis, testes, scrotum, and prostate gland.

At the 6th week of pregnancy it is impossible to tell the difference between a boy and girl, but by the 12th week a male foetus will have started to develop a penis and testicles in a scrotal sac. By the time a baby is born, both testicles should have descended into the scrotal sac outside the body.

During puberty, the penis is the fastest growing part of the body. The average adult penis is 7.5–10cm (3–4in) when flaccid and 15–17.5cm (6–7in) long when it's erect. During puberty it's quite normal for a boy to have as many as 20 reflex erections a day. As adults, many men still continue to have four or five erections during a night's sleep.

The prostate gland is the size of a walnut and sits just below the bladder. Its main function is to store and secrete fluid that forms part of semen. It also contains muscle fibres which help to expel semen during ejaculation.

SEMEN AND SPERM

Semen is made up of sperm and secretions from the seminal vesicles, prostate, and other glands in the genital tract. Normal semen is clear or white; a yellow tinge may suggest infection, and pink or brown could mean it contains blood. This may simply be caused by vigorous sexual intercourse or overzealous masturbation, but you should talk to your doctor. When first produced, semen is thick and slightly sticky but then becomes watery within a few minutes of ejaculation. Normal volumes range from 2–6ml (0.3–1tsps) and normally there are around 20 million sperm in each millilitre.

WHAT DOES AN ABNORMAL SEMEN ANALYSIS MEAN?

About one in 20 men has an abnormal semen analysis. This can mean a low sperm count, abnormal sperm, or sperm that are not as mobile as they should be.

If the sperm count is low, you may be able to improve it. Sperm are made in your testes and production is at its

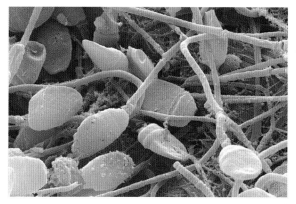

▲ Each sperm has a head containing the genetic material and a long, whip-like tail used to propel the sperm.

best if your testes are cool. Doctors advise men with low counts to wear loose-fitting clothes: wear boxer shorts rather than Y-fronts and avoid tight jeans. Hot baths are not recommended, and cycling is best avoided as it prevents cooling air circulation. Smoking and drinking alcohol also reduce sperm counts. So stop smoking and stick to 16 units of alcohol (or fewer) each week. Don't ejaculate more than once a day, as too much sex can reduce the sperm in each ejaculate.

Some prescription medicines and street drugs such as cannabis and cocaine can also reduce your sperm count. But never stop taking a prescription medication without first talking to your doctor. He or she may be able to suggest an alternative if your medication has got the side effect of reducing the sperm count.

WHAT IF I NOTICE BLOOD IN MY SEMEN?

Called haemospermia, blood in the semen can affect men of any age. It is rarely due to anything serious but you should still get it checked out by your doctor to be sure, particularly if you are over 40. In fact, most cases turn out to be due to nothing more than enthusiastic sex or masturbation.

HOW SAFE IS WITHDRAWAL AS A METHOD OF CONTRACEPTION?

Not safe enough! Even if you are 100 per cent reliable in using the withdrawal method, there are sperm in the secretions that leak from your penis prior to ejaculation, and it only takes one sperm! Always use a more reliable form of contraception.

DR DAWN'S HEALTH CHECK
Giving a semen sample

Most semen samples are analysed to assess the quality and quantity of sperm so they need to be produced in ideal circumstances to ensure the sperm remain as healthy as possible.

In practice, this means that a sample has to be produced by masturbation after two or three days with no ejaculation. Soap and lubricants should not be used immediately beforehand as these may be toxic to the sperm. The entire ejaculate should be collected directly into the container. It must be kept warm and delivered to the laboratory for testing within a couple of hours.

If it will be difficult for you to deliver the sample within this time limit, speak to your doctor as he or she will be able to arrange for you to produce a sample at the laboratory.

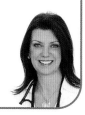

IMPOTENCE

Impotence, or erectile dysfunction as doctors call it, is far more common than you think. It affects most men at some point but it's a recurring problem for as many as one in ten men over 30, and you shouldn't ignore it. Aside from the fact that it often divides relationships, it can be the first sign that your arteries are furred up (see Coronary heart disease p.52).

WHAT YOU CAN DO

If you have persistent problems, you should see your doctor. You need to have your blood pressure checked, and you should have blood tests to assess your cholesterol level and to rule out diabetes. If all your tests are normal, then making a few adjustments to lifestyle may help. Smoking, drinking to excess, being overweight, using street drugs such as cannabis or cocaine, or taking anabolic steroids can all cause impotence. And there's stress and guilt, which may be more difficult to deal with but play a significant role.

DRUGS FOR IMPOTENCE

The launch of medication such as sildenafil (better known by its brand name Viagra) has revolutionized the

▼ Impotence affects most men at some point; talking about it with your partner may forestall relationship problems.

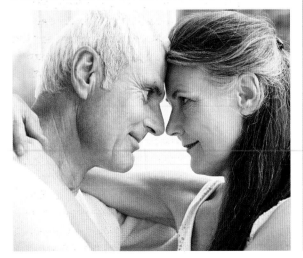

treatment of impotence. But don't be tempted just to buy them on the Internet – they can interact with other drugs so you need to talk to your doctor about them; believe me, your doctor will have heard it all before so there's no need for embarrassment.

DR DAWN'S HEALTH CHECK

Is there such a thing as the male menopause?

Strictly speaking, men can't have a menopause, as the word actually means cessation of periods. Men don't experience a sudden loss of the male hormone testosterone in the same way that women lose oestrogen. However, some men do suffer from the effects of a steady decline in their testosterone levels, so yes, I think the male menopause does exist but perhaps we should call it the "andropause".

Low testosterone levels can be associated with a loss of sex drive, difficulty achieving or maintaining an erection, weight gain, depression, anxiety, fatigue, and even shrinking testicles. But we must be careful not to medicalize the male midlife crisis. It is normal for anyone to take stock of their life after 40, let alone 50, to reassess what they want in the future. However, if you run off with a younger woman, low testosterone levels are not the explanation!

Is there a male HRT?

Yes there is. Men with confirmed low levels of testosterone can have replacement in the form of patches or gels, but it's not without risks. Testosterone can raise levels of bad cholesterol, possibly increasing the risk of heart disease, and may also increase the risk of developing prostate cancer (see p.160). A better option is probably to watch your alcohol intake and keep fit; fit men have higher testosterone levels than men who are not active.

FIND OUT MORE
www.malehealth.co.uk

PENIS PROBLEMS

Many men have problems with their penis at some point. Probably the most common concern is impotence (see left) but there are lots of other things that can go wrong.

BALANITIS

Balanitis is inflammation of the head (glans) of the penis. It is most commonly due to infection with a fungus or bacteria and can usually be easily treated with antibiotic or antifungal creams or tablets. It can happen to any man but those with a foreskin that is difficult to pull back and men who don't wash thoroughly enough around the glans are more at risk, as are diabetics.

PHIMOSIS

Phimosis is due to a tight band of inelastic skin at the tip of the foreskin that prevents it from retracting fully. It is common in young boys and can usually be treated with steroid creams and gentle daily stretching. Most cases clear up by the age of four without needing surgery. Persistent phimosis in adults is more likely to require surgery – either a slit in the foreskin or circumcision.

DR DAWN'S HEALTH CHECK
Circumcision

Circumcision is the surgical removal of all or part of the foreskin. In the UK, about one in 20 men is circumcised. The operation causes temporary soreness, which can generally be controlled with simple painkillers.

What are the pros and cons?
There is evidence that urinary tract infections, syphilis, herpes, and HIV infection are less common in circumcised men. However, circumcised men are more likely to suffer from genital warts, gonorrhoea and nongonoccoal urethritis (NGU). Bottom line? I wouldn't put my boys through circumcision without good reason. There is also evidence that circumcised men have reduced sensation, but circumcision has not been shown to help sufferers of premature ejaculation and it's not an option I would recommend.

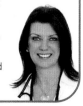

PARAPHIMOSIS

Paraphimosis occurs when the foreskin is stuck behind the glans and then starts to restrict blood flow. The foreskin should be gently eased back over the glans as soon as possible; if you can't manage it at home, seek medical advice – in the worse case, paraphimosis that is left could cause gangrene of the penis.

PEYRONIE'S DISEASE

This condition causes a bend in the erect penis. In its mildest form, it produces a minimal curve that doesn't usually cause too many problems, but more severe disease can produce such marked angulation that makes penetrative sex difficult or even impossible.

Treatment depends upon the severity. Mild cases may not need treatment. In severe cases, surgery may be suggested but this causes slight shortening of the penis, and since up to one in five cases clears up by itself within 18 months, it's not an option to rush into.

FIND OUT MORE
www.malehealth.co.uk

PROSTATE ENLARGEMENT

The prostate gland is a small, walnut-shaped gland that sits just below the bladder. The urethra (the tube that takes urine from the bladder through the penis to the outside) runs through the prostate. It is normal for the prostate to enlarge with age, causing many men over 50 to have problems with urinating.

BENIGN PROSTATIC HYPERTROPHY (BPH)

The prostate starts to enlarge in middle age – about one third of 50-year-olds have some degree of enlargement – and because it's the central part of the gland that tends to grow, it often causes pressure on the urethra and difficulties with passing urine. As its name implies, BPH is not cancerous. The problem is that the symptoms of benign disease and prostate cancer are similar so should always be checked by your doctor. In particular, you

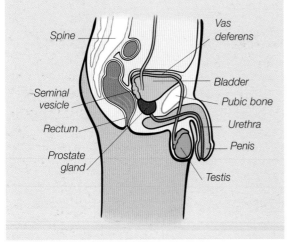

▲ *Organs of the male reproductive system.*

should see your doctor if you develop:

• Hesitancy (difficulty in starting to urinate) and/or the need to strain to urinate.

• A weak stream.

• The feeling that your bladder isn't empty after urination.

• The need to pass urine urgently and/or frequently.

• The need to get up at night more than once to urinate.

• A burning sensation or pain when passing urine.

• Blood in your urine.

Your doctor will ask you questions about your urine flow and will then want to perform a digital rectal examination, which involves inserting a finger into the rectum to feel the size of the gland.

TREATMENT FOR BPH

As long as there is no cancer, it is safe to wait and see. Some cases improve without treatment, but in just over half the problem gets worse and treatment may be sought. In the first instance, men with BPH will be offered medication that shrinks the prostate. Otherwise, there is an operation called TURP (transurethral resection of prostate), in which the central part of the prostate is removed – a bit like coring an apple.

FIND OUT MORE
www.malehealth.co.uk

PROSTATE CANCER

Excluding skin cancer, prostate cancer is the most common cancer in the world and accounts for seven out of ten cancers in men. However, many of the cancers grow so slowly that men die with the cancer not because of it. Most men over the age of 80 have prostate cancer at autopsy, but only four per cent actually die of it.

WHAT ARE THE SYMPTOMS?

Passing urine more frequently, having to get up at night to urinate, a hesitancy before you urinate, or a weak stream can all be symptoms of prostate disease. However, these symptoms do not necessarily mean cancer; benign (noncancerous) enlargement of the prostate – known as benign prostatic hypertrophy (BPH, see previous article) – can also cause these symptoms. If you have any of the symptoms, you should see your doctor and get some tests to make sure.

HOW IS IT DIAGNOSED AND TREATED?

Your doctor will question you about your symptoms, particularly urinary symptoms, and will probably want to carry out a digital rectal examination to check the size of your prostate gland. This examination involves inserting a finger into the rectum; it may be uncomfortable but shouldn't be painful. Your doctor may also take a blood sample for a PSA test.

? **DID YOU KNOW**
Who is at risk?

• Having a first degree relative (brother, father, or son) with prostate cancer doubles your likelihood of developing the disease.

• Increasing age is another important factor – men under the age of 40 have a one in 10,000 risk, but this rises to one in eight if you are over the age of 60.

• Ethnicity plays a role too, with African men being at greatest risk.

• Research from Australia suggests that men who ejaculate the most frequently are the least likely to develop prostate cancer.

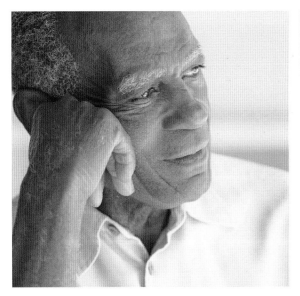

▲ *Prostate cancer is one of the most common cancers. It mainly affects older men but is rarely fatal.*

This test checks for levels of a chemical called prostate specific antigen (PSA) in your blood. However, it isn't as reliable as doctors had hoped. The PSA levels are normal in 20 per cent of prostate cancers and up to three-quarters of men with raised levels don't have cancer but have BPH. For this reason, I am not keen on routine PSA testing in the absence of other symptoms. Personally, I think the PSA test should be offered to men with symptoms of prostate disease, a family history of the cancer, and those who have an enlarged prostate found on rectal examination.

If the test results indicate that prostate cancer is a possibility, you will be given a prostate biopsy, an uncomfortable procedure in which a sample of prostate tissue is removed for analysis. If cancer is confirmed, treatment may be offered.

Treatment options vary according to your age, general health, and how far advanced the cancer is. You may be offered surgery, which carries the risk of incontinence and impotence, radiotherapy, or medication. Sometimes, no treatment is the best option.

TESTICULAR CANCER

Overall, testicular cancer is rare, although it is one of the commoner forms of cancer diagnosed in younger men. The good news is that it's also one of the most easily cured if it is found at an early stage. All men should make a point of checking their testicles from puberty onwards so that they know what is normal for them and can report any changes.

HOW TO CHECK YOUR TESTICLES

The best way to do this is in a warm shower when the muscle in the scrotal sac is relaxed. It is normal, for example, to have one testicle larger than the other and for one to hang down slightly lower.

Hold your scrotum gently in the palms of your hands and, using your fingers and thumbs, feel each testicle individually. If you do this regularly, it'll be obvious if any lumps develop. If you find a new lump, get it checked by your doctor straight away. Most lumps turn out to be non-cancerous cysts, but there are around 2,000 cases of testicular cancer in the UK each year and, unlike most cancers, testicular cancer can strike young – many cancers are in men under the age of 30.

TREATMENT

Most cases of testicular cancer are curable with surgery and chemotherapy. If the cancer is caught early, surgery alone gives a 99 per cent cure rate, but given that in about one third of all new diagnoses the cancer has already spread from the testicle, chemotherapy is often needed as well. Amazingly, even then the cure rate is still around 95 per cent. So the message is, quite literally, don't die of embarrassment – check yourself regularly and report any changes to your doctor straight away.

FIND OUT MORE
www.prostate-cancer.org.uk

FIND OUT MORE
www.orchid-cancer.org.uk

• Having sex at least twice a week helps to boost the immune system, and may ward off the common cold • Most men ejaculate within two minutes of penetration • Testosterone levels peak between 7a.m. and 9a.m. and reach their lowest in the late afternoon • Sexual intercourse expends similar energy levels to climbing two flights of stairs • One in six British holiday makers under 30 has sex with a new partner while on holiday and only half use a condom • People who have regular sex live longer.

15

Sexual health & fertility

Introduction We are living in a rapidly changing world when it comes to sex. In the 1960s, only one in 100 women had had sex under the age of 16. Today the figure is closer to one in four. Most British youngsters will have lost their virginity by the age of 20, and there is no doubt that the number of sexual partners any one person has is also on the increase. Add to that the continuing rise in divorce (meaning more older adults are looking for a sexual partner, and they may be less comfortable with the concept of carrying their own condoms), and it is easy to see why sexually transmitted infections are on the increase.

It is very important to remember that sexually transmitted infections are not fussy. If you are have unprotected sex, you are at risk. They really couldn't care if you are posh, rich, or even famous – wear a condom! And remember HIV is not just a gay issue, it affects heterosexuals too, and it is still very much out there.

LIBIDO

I see a lot of people in the surgery concerned that they have lost their sex drive. Most are looking for an underlying medical problem to explain their loss of libido, and of course sometimes there are medical causes, but usually it is due to emotional and psychological factors rather than physical illness.

WHAT ABOUT TESTOSTERONE REPLACEMENT?

Testosterone levels affect a person's libido and, yes, women produce it too, although in smaller amounts than men. Half a woman's testosterone is produced in her ovaries. A study in the United States showed that women who experienced a loss of libido after their ovaries had been removed benefited from testosterone replacement in the form of a patch. Testosterone is not licensed for this use in the UK, and it isn't without its problems either. Side effects include acne, increased facial hair, and depression – hardly likely to make a woman feel particularly sexy.

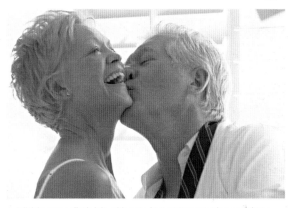

▲ *Libido may diminish with age but many couples continue to have pleasurable sex well into old age – the trick is good communication and accommodating each other's needs.*

DR DAWN'S HEALTH CHECK
Loss of interest in sex

If you have lost interest in sex, ask yourself some questions:
• Are you tired?
It is only human to consider your bed to be a place for sleeping if you are exhausted. New parents often find the responsibility of a baby and endless sleepless nights result in reduced sex drive, and this is normal. Rest assured, your sex drive will come back but don't be surprised if it takes up to a year. Tiredness can also be related to physical problems, such as anaemia or thyroid disease, so it's worth seeing your doctor for some simple tests.
• Are you depressed?
Feeling tired all the time or having no interest in sex can be the early signs of depression. If this could be you, make an appointment to see your doctor.
• Do you feel attractive?
Women particularly find that feeling less attractive has an adverse effect on their sex drive and weight gain is the most common culprit. If you take regular exercise, it actually boosts your energy levels and helps with your weight, which is bound to make you feel better about yourself.
• Do you still find your partner attractive?
There is so much more to attraction than physical appearance. But if your six-pack rugby player has turned into a couch potato, or after three children your blushing bride has gained as many stones, then you may not find each other as attractive. This can be difficult to admit to yourself and even more difficult to talk about, but working on a healthy living programme together may be the answer.
• Do you resent your partner?
If deep down you want to rip your husband's head off for never helping with the children's bedtime or you feel deeply angry that your wife is spending money like wildfire, then it is hardly surprising that you don't feel like making love. Resentment is a difficult emotion to deal with. Try to be honest with your partner about how you feel. If you come to an impasse of mutual criticism, counselling as a couple may help you to see each other's point of view and remember the good points that brought you together in the first place.
• Are you on any medication?
Lots of medicines can affect libido, but be honest with yourself – has the problem only started since taking new medication? If the answer is yes, then talk to your doctor; there will almost certainly be a better alternative. However, never stop taking a prescribed drug without consulting your doctor.

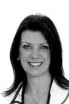

ALCOHOL AND SEX

Does alcohol give Dutch courage or brewer's droop? Alcohol depresses the central nervous system and as such can help you to relax when you are anxious. But when it comes to sex, it can affect your judgement and your inhibitions.

EFFECT ON WOMEN

A couple of units of alcohol (a unit is a small glass of wine or a single measure of spirits, see p.77) can reduce your inhibitions and enhance your sexual desire, but beware – alcohol also impairs your judgement. Sexual arousal affects your judgement too and the combination can easily lead to unprotected sex and the possibility of contracting sexually transmitted diseases or becoming pregnant. Alcohol can also reduce your sexual response, and chronic alcohol intake will reduce your libido.

EFFECT ON MEN

Alcohol can also have a negative effect on men – even a small amount can cause temporary erectile failure. It can also cause delayed ejaculation. Some of my male patients have used it as a self-help treatment for premature ejaculation, but there's a fine line so be careful.

   In the longterm, chronic heavy alcohol use is associated with low testosterone levels, which in turn causes problems with reduced libido, impotence, reduced ejaculate, and poor-quality sperm.

▼ Alcohol can reduce inhibitions and increase desire but tends to impair judgement and sexual response.

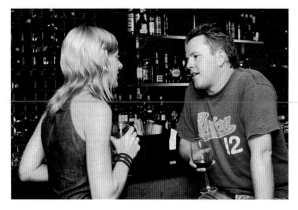

BENIGN COITAL HEADACHE

About one person in 100 suffers from a condition called benign coital headache. The headache starts as orgasm is reached and lasts 15–20 minutes. Coital headache is more common in men than women and anyone who gets migraines is also at increased risk. The good news is that the headaches don't persist – most people find they return to a headache-free sex life after a while without the need for medical treatment.

WHAT YOU CAN DO

Before you are likely to have sex, try taking a painkiller such as ibuprofen or paracetamol. If this doesn't work and the headaches continue to cause problems, it's worth seeing your doctor.

   Your doctor will probably check your blood pressure, as coital headaches can be associated with high blood pressure. He or she may prescribe a beta-blocker drug normally used to treat recurrent migraines or high blood pressure as studies have shown it helps in persistent coital headaches.

VAGINISMUS

This occurs when the muscles around the entrance to the vagina go into spasm as soon as your partner tries to enter, making penetrative sex impossible. In extreme cases, it happens when you try to use a tampon or insert a finger into your vagina.

CAUSES AND TREATMENT

Vaginismus is almost always psychological in origin and, as a result, anxiety about the condition will make it worse. The good news is that psychosexual counselling really can help to cure the problem and the success rates are as high as 80 per cent, so don't be afraid to seek medical advice if you are affected.

CONTRACEPTION

Most sexual activity is for pleasure and not procreation and with that comes an obvious need for contraception. Whole books have been written about contraception and sadly there isn't the space in a book like this to cover every option in detail, but I hope I can give you an idea of what is available and where you can go for more advice.

WHAT ARE THE OPTIONS?

There is more contraceptive choice today than ever before so let's take a quick look at what is available:

• The condom – an excellent form of contraception (up to 98 per cent effective if used properly) that also protects against many sexually transmitted infections. Make sure you always use ones with the British Standard kitemark or the European CE marking. The best are those containing the spermicide nonoxinol-9. If you are using condoms, avoid oil-based lubricants such as massage oils or petroleum jelly as they can weaken the rubber.

• The female condom – this is a one-size female condom that can be inserted into the vagina. It works, but most women I have met who have tried it liken it to making love through a crisp packet!

• Caps and diaphragms – these can be placed in the vagina several hours before sex so you need not interrupt lovemaking. They are quoted as being up to 96 per cent effective but this does rely on their being used properly, which some women find tricky. In my opinion, they are a great form of contraception for anyone not wanting to use hormones but for whom pregnancy wouldn't be a disaster.

▼ The combined oral contraceptive pill (COC) is reliable and is the most popular choice of contraception.

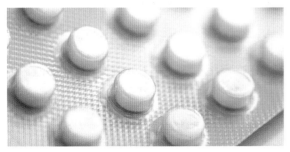

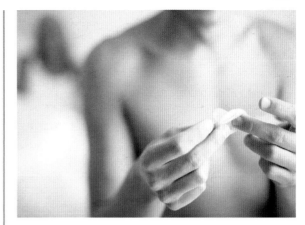

▲ The male condom is up to 98 per cent effective and also helps protect against sexually transmitted infections.

• The pill – this usually means the combined contraceptive pill (COC), which contains both oestrogen and progestogen. It works predominantly by stopping ovulation. There are lots of brands available, containing different amounts of oestrogen and progestogen, so if you don't get on with one then ask your doctor about an alternative. The COC isn't for everyone, though, and you shouldn't take it if you:

  • Have a family history of blood clots.
  • Have high blood pressure.
  • Are over 35 and smoke.
  • Are severely obese (BMI over 39).
  • Have known liver disease.
  • Have migraine with aura.
  • Are pregnant or breastfeeding.
  • Have breast cancer.

Side effects such as bloating, breast tenderness, mood swings, weight gain, and headaches are common in the early stages of use but tend to disappear with time.

• The patch – like the pill, the patch contains both oestrogen and progestogen so has similar side effects and cautions. The patch only needs replacing every week so is a good option for anyone who finds taking a pill every day difficult to remember.

• The minipill – also known as the progestogen-only pill (POP), this is an excellent alternative for women who can't take oestrogen. Unlike the COC, it really must be taken at the same time or within three hours of that time every day (with the exception of one of the newer brands, which must be taken within 12 hours) and

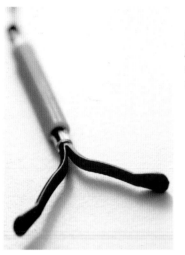

◀ *The IUS is placed in the uterus and provides effective contraception for five years.*

instead of giving a regular light bleed, some women find they have erratic bleeding using the POP. Common side effects include weight gain, breast tenderness, and spotty skin.

• The injection – there are two contraceptive injections used in the UK. They are given every eight or 12 weeks, usually into the buttock. They contain just progestogen and are particularly useful for women who forget to take pills. They can cause erratic bleeding and, although they have no long-term effect on fertility, unlike other progestogen-only methods, it can take up to a year for fertility to return completely to normal, so contraceptive injections are best avoided by women planning a family in the near future. There has also been concern about their effect on bone mass and, although there is no proven link between their use and the development of osteoporosis later in life, I am cautious about using them in women who are at high risk of osteoporosis.

• The implant – another progestogen-only method, this is a small rod the size of a matchstick that is inserted (under local anaesthetic) beneath the skin in the upper arm. It needs to be replaced after three years.

• The intra-uterine system (IUS) – this is a small, T-shaped device that is placed in the uterus and secretes tiny amounts of progestogen (about the same as two minipills a week) directly where it is needed – the uterine lining. It may cause erratic bleeding for a few months but most women find the bleeding settles and many stop their periods altogether after six months. The IUS needs to be replaced every five years.

• The coil – this looks similar to the IUS but does not contain any hormone. There are several brands available, lasting anything up to 10 years. They are very effective but shouldn't be used by women at high risk of sexually transmitted infection or ectopic pregnancy. Some women find their periods are heavier using the coil but since many women go from using the pill, which tends to cause lighter periods, to using a coil, they are not necessarily comparing like with like.

WHAT ABOUT THE "MORNING AFTER PILL"?

The "morning after pill" is something of a misnomer as it implies that it must be taken the following morning. In fact, it can be taken anything up to 72 hours after unprotected sex, although the earlier the better. It does not require a doctor's prescription and can be bought over the counter at pharmacies; many "out of hours" centres also carry a stock.

WHERE CAN I GO FOR CONTRACEPTION?

Your doctor can prescribe pills and patches and give injections. Many can also fit coils, implants, and the intra-uterine system. If you don't want to see your family doctor, you can actually see any GP for contraceptive services (you don't have to be registered at the practice) or you can make your own appointment at your local family planning clinic; to find your nearest clinic (and for more information about contraceptive choices), visit the website at the bottom of this page.

The contraceptive implant is a matchstick-sized rod inserted under the skin in the upper arm. ▶

FIND OUT MORE
www.fpa.org.uk

SEXUALLY TRANSMITTED INFECTIONS

If you remember nothing else about sexually transmitted infections (STIs), remember this: they are not fussy – they can infect anybody who is sexually active. Believe me, the nicest people can and do contract STIs, so if you are having sex with a new partner, always use a condom. Remember, when you have sex with someone, you are also, in effect, having sex with everyone that person has ever had sex with.

CHECK IT OUT

Some STIs are obvious – you will notice a discharge or blisters – but there may be no symptoms at all, so your partner may have no idea he or she is putting you at risk.

If you are concerned that you may have an STI and don't want to see your own doctor, you can go to any genitourinary medicine clinic. It doesn't even have to be the one nearest to your home.

CHLAMYDIA

This disease is transmitted by penetrative or oral sex and is so common that as many as one in eight young sexually active people have the infection. However, 70–90 per cent of infected women and 50 per cent of all infected men have no symptoms and therefore continue to unwittingly put new partners at risk. If left untreated, chlamydia can cause pelvic inflammatory disease in women and it's the main preventable cause of infertility. In men, chlamydia is the main cause of nongonococcal urethritis (NGU).

Chlamydia is easily diagnosed with a simple swab or urine test, and it can be effectively treated with antibiotics, so don't ignore the risks. If you have had unprotected sex, get yourself tested.

GONORRHOEA

This often causes a vaginal or penile discharge but, as with chlamydia, there may not be any symptoms – around half of all infected women have no symptoms. Again, it is easily diagnosed with a swab test and can be treated with antibiotics.

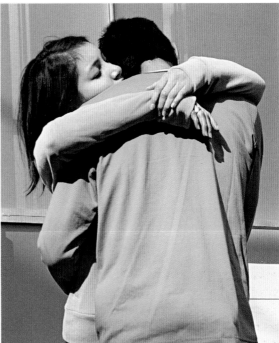

▲ *A sexually transmitted infection won't necessarily cause any symptoms and can infect anybody who is sexually active.*

HERPES

This condition is caused by a virus and is spread by skin-to-skin contact, so you don't need to be having penetrative sex to be at risk and a condom won't give you complete protection. About 70 per cent of people infected with the virus have no symptoms. When there are symptoms, they typically develop 7–10 days after contact with the virus; the main symptom is painful sores in the genital region but there may also be pain when passing urine and, in women, a vaginal discharge.

Once in your body the herpes virus never completely clears so once you are infected, you could have recurrent attacks. However, symptoms tend to be less severe in subsequent attacks, and the time between attacks usually increases. You should not have sex while symptoms are present.

Antiviral drugs prescribed by your doctor can reduce the severity and duration of an attack, but as yet there is no complete cure. This is why it is important to remember that even if you have no symptoms, you can still pass on the infection.

GENITAL WARTS

Warts on the genitals, like other warts, are caused by the human papillomavirus (HPV). Only one in ten people carrying the virus develops visible warts – half will develop them within three months of acquiring the virus but the other half may not notice any warts for several years. I have seen many relationships suffer under the assumption that a partner must have been unfaithful when in fact he or she could have contracted the virus from a relationship years before. The warts are usually soft, with a rough surface, and are painless. They tend to grow rapidly and sometimes cluster together. Some genital warts are linked to cancer of the cervix and anus but, interestingly, the more florid and ugly the warts, the less likely they are to be associated with cancer.

Genital warts are treated by painting them with several applications of special medicated paints to remove them. The risk of acquiring them can be reduced by using safer sex practices (see box opposite), although condoms do not give complete protection, and it is advisable to avoid sex when the warts are visible.

DR DAWN'S HEALTH CHECK
When you should see a doctor

Genitourinary medicine clinics across the UK diagnosed nearly 800,000 new cases of sexually transmitted infections in 2006. And according to one British survey, one in nine men and one in eight women aged 16–44 reported having had an STI at some point. STIs are common and don't care how clean or smart you or your partner are – if you are having sex, you are potentially putting yourself at risk.

So the message is simple: don't let embarrassment stand in your way – you should see a doctor if you have unprotected sex with a new partner, whether or not you or your new partner develop symptoms.

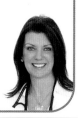

FIND OUT MORE
www.fpa.org.uk
www.playingsafely.co.uk

HIV INFECTION

HIV (human immunodeficiency virus) can be passed between people in several ways – sex is just one of them. It can be transferred in blood, semen and pre-ejaculate fluids, and vaginal and menstrual fluids. HIV can also be passed from an infected mother to her baby in the uterus, during childbirth, or in breast milk. Thankfully, it is now very rare in the UK for babies to be infected with HIV because HIV-positive mothers are given special medical care during pregnancy and childbirth, and they and their babies also receive special care after the birth.

WHO IS AT RISK?

The main groups at risk are those who:

- Have unprotected sex (anal, vaginal, or oral) with someone infected with HIV.
- Share sex toys with an infected person.
- Share needles with an infected person.
- Receive a blood transfusion in a country that doesn't screen for HIV infection. (All blood donors in the UK are routinely screened for HIV so this doesn't apply here.)

Hugging, sharing cups, plates, cutlery, and toilet seats are all safe. In theory, prolonged kissing with an open mouth if you have a cut could pose a risk, but to all intents and purposes kissing is considered safe.

CAN YOU CATCH HIV THROUGH ORAL SEX?

Yes, although the risks are much lower than via anal or vaginal sex and the risk is mainly to anyone performing oral sex on an infected man. There is little evidence to show that HIV is passed on when performing oral sex on a woman. You can reduce your risks by:

- Always using a condom during oral sex.
- Avoiding oral sex when you have a sore throat or cuts or abrasions in your mouth.
- Cleaning and flossing your teeth before oral sex. However, you should make sure you don't accidentally make your gums bleed. If you do, then you should avoid oral sex.
- Avoiding getting pre-ejaculate or semen in your mouth.
- Avoiding oral sex during a woman's period.

HOW WOULD I KNOW IF I HAVE CAUGHT HIV?

To be honest, unless you have a test, you probably wouldn't. As many as half those infected don't get any symptoms in the early stages. Some people develop a mild flu-like illness a few days or weeks after infection. The illness usually lasts for one or two weeks but as the symptoms are vague and mild, they are often ignored.

IF I KNOW I AM AT RISK, HOW SOON CAN I HAVE A TEST AFTER SEX?

When you are infected with HIV, your body will start producing antibodies to the virus but it can take up to three months before there are enough antibodies to show up in a blood test.

WHERE CAN I HAVE AN HIV TEST?

Most GP surgeries will arrange an HIV test for you but if you would rather not use your family doctor, you can arrange to have the test done at a family planning, genitourinary medicine (GUM), or sexual health clinic.

WHAT HAPPENS IF I HAVE A POSITIVE TEST?

A positive test means you have been infected with the virus. No test is 100 per cent reliable and you may be offered a second blood test to confirm the result. If this is still positive, you will be referred to a specialist for further tests to check how the virus has affected your immune system and to decide whether or not you need to start

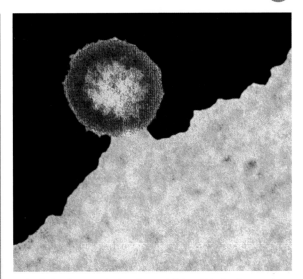

▲ *A photomicrograph showing an HIV particle (red) emerging from a human cell (green).*

treatment. A positive test result is obviously difficult to come to terms with but it is vital that you share the result with any sexual partners so that they can be tested too.

IS THERE A CURE FOR HIV?

At the moment, there is no cure for the virus but there are effective drugs that treat many of the conditions associated with HIV infection, and antiretroviral drugs that seem to help reduce the level of virus in the blood and delay the onset of AIDS

HOW LONG DOES IT TAKE TO DEVELOP AIDS IF YOU ARE HIV-POSITIVE?

That's a bit like asking how long is a piece of string? Some people become ill with full-blown AIDS within a few weeks of having a positive test (although they may have had the virus for months or years without knowing). Others can live for 20 years before developing signs of AIDS. Make sure you attend your regular check-ups to monitor the disease, and look after your immune system by eating healthily, exercising regularly, and keeping stress to a minimum.

DR DAWN'S HEALTH CHECK

Safer sex practices

You can reduce your chances of contracting an STI by:

• Reducing the number of sexual partners you have.

• Talking openly to anyone you may have sex with before your judgement is lost in a moment of passion.

• Watching your alcohol intake – lost inhibitions have put several people in my clinic room on a Monday morning!

• Carrying condoms with you, and using them.

• Using a dental dam for oral sex (the end of a condom makes a good DIY dam).

• Covering sex toys with a condom.

• Not letting anyone persuade you that if they withdraw before ejaculating you'll be safe. The pre-ejaculation fluid can contain sperm and organisms that cause STIs.

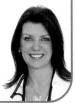

FIND OUT MORE
www.tht.org.uk

FERTILITY

In around 90 per cent of couples trying to conceive, the woman becomes pregnant within 12 months, and in another five per cent the woman becomes pregnant within two years, leaving five in every 100 couples who fail to conceive despite regular intercourse. In some couples, all the medical tests doctors carry out come back normal and we simply don't know why they can't get pregnant, but in most instances we can identify a problem.

COMMON CAUSES OF INFERTILITY

The most common causes are:

- Abnormal sperm – in about 30 per cent of cases.
- Failure to ovulate – in about 25 per cent of cases.
- Damaged fallopian tubes from previous infection – in about 20 per cent of cases.
- Endometriosis – in about 5 per cent of cases.

WHEN IS THE BEST TIME FOR SEX IF YOU WANT TO CONCEIVE?

Sexual intercourse around the time of ovulation is most likely to result in a pregnancy. Women ovulate 14 days before the start of the next period. If you have a regular cycle, it is easy to predict when you ovulate. There are also ovulation predictor kits available, but I'm not keen on them. They predict ovulation reliably but, surprisingly, their use doesn't seem to improve the chance of conception and can cause a great deal of anxiety.

WHEN SHOULD YOU SEE YOUR DOCTOR?

This depends on your age. If you are 20, you have time on your side and, given that 95 per cent of couples conceive within two years, it is reasonable to keep trying for a couple of years before seeking help. If, on the other hand, you are 35 and have had no luck after about six months, then it's probably time to talk things through with your doctor.

WHAT TESTS WILL THE DOCTOR DO?

The first tests I do on a couple who are having difficulty conceiving are a semen analysis on the man and a blood test on the woman.

The man should not have ejaculated for at least two days before producing the sample and it should be collected directly into a sterile container, not via a condom, because some condoms are impregnated with spermicide, which would adversely affect the result. The woman's blood test needs to be taken on day 21 of the

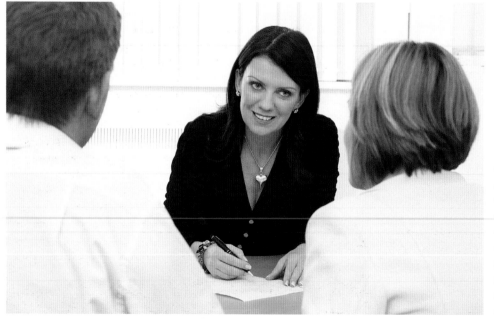

◄ *Young couples who have difficulty conceiving should probably see their doctor after about a couple of years of trying. For older couples, it's advisable to get medical advice sooner, after about six months.*

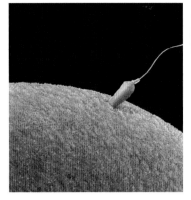

A photomicrograph showing a sperm fertilizing an egg. ▶

menstrual cycle (counting day one as the first day of her last period). The test is looking for a rise in the level of the hormone progesterone, which indicates ovulation. A low level suggests a woman hasn't ovulated that cycle, although it doesn't necessarily mean she never ovulates so it's worth repeating the test on two or three cycles. I would also check levels of other hormones, thyroid function, and for chlamydia antibodies. If the chlamydia antibody test is strongly positive, it is possible that the woman's fallopian tubes have been damaged as a result of chlamydia infection, and she may need to be referred to a specialist to see if the tubes are blocked.

DR DAWN'S HEALTH CHECK
How to improve your fertility

• Stay positive – one in four couples go to their doctor to discuss fertility and the majority will ultimately have a child.
• Have intercourse only every two to three days.
• If you smoke, give up.
• Keep your alcohol intake within recommended limits.
• Don't use any recreational drugs.
• Men should keep their testicles cool – no tight jeans or hot baths.
• Women need to maintain a healthy body weight (your BMI should be between 18.5 and 24.9, see p.94).

? DID YOU KNOW
What treatment is there for infertility?

The treatment you need depends on why you are having problems conceiving. If you are not ovulating, we can try to kick-start your ovaries with a drug called clomifene. If you have endometriosis, laser treatment can help and is the only endometriosis treatment proven to improve fertility. If your fallopian tubes are blocked, your specialist may suggest surgery to try to open them, although sadly the results of this sort of surgery are not that good.

Low sperm production due to an underactive thyroid gland can be treated with replacement hormones. However, underactivity of the thyroid is a very rare cause of male infertility and so this treatment is simply not applicable for the vast majority of infertile men.

All the treatments above are available on the NHS but if you need assisted conception, which is very expensive, then you'll probably have to fund it yourself. Some Primary Care Trusts (PCTs) offer eligible couples one assisted conception attempt but many do not offer it at all. Your doctor can tell you what's available in your area.

Types of assisted conception
The main types of assisted conception are:
• IVF (in vitro fertilization) – this involves putting an egg and sperm together in a test tube to produce an embryo. Usually the woman will require drugs to stimulate her ovaries. The eggs are then removed, fertilized, and replaced. There is about a 20 per cent chance of a successful pregnancy.
• GIFT (gamete intrafallopian transfer) – this involves placing an egg and the sperm directly into the fallopian tube. It will only work if the tubes are healthy, and it has a similar success rate to IVF.
• ICSI (intracytoplasmic sperm injection) – this is used for male infertility or for couples who have been unsuccessful with IVF and involves injecting a single sperm into a single egg with similar success rates as IVF.
• Egg donation – useful for women who have had a premature menopause or are unsuccessful with IVF.
• Sperm donation – if the man has no sperm at all or a very poor count, this may be the only option.

FIND OUT MORE
www.fpa.org.uk

• The human brain contains over 100 billion nerves, and each one is linked to 10,000 others • Nerve fibres vary in length, from microscopic to over 1 metre (3ft) long • Over half the cells in our nervous system do not actually transmit any impulses. They are there simply to support the active cells • Your spinal cord is about the same width as your thumb for most of its length • Nerve impulses fire off twice as quickly in adults as they do in newborn infants • Normal adult nerve impulses travel back to the brain at over 250km/h (155m/h).

16

Neurological & mental health

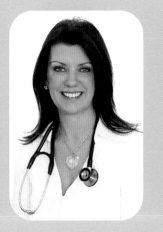

Introduction The human body is governed by the nervous system. This system consists of over 100,000 million nerve cells, each one with around 10,000 connections, making it the most complicated machine in the world. The system is comprised of the central nervous system – your brain and spinal cord; the peripheral nervous system – the nerves that supply the different parts of your body; and the automatic nervous system – that controls functions not under conscious control, such as heart rate and breathing.

The average brain weighs 1.4kg (3lb). Its surface is covered by a thin layer called the cerebral cortex, which if spread out flat would cover $1m^2$ ($1yd^2$). Twelve pairs of cranial nerves come directly from the brain to the head and face. The spinal cord is about 45cm (18in) long and sprouts 31 pairs of nerves, ultimately responsible for movement, coordination, and sensations of touch, pain, vibration, and temperature.

The interaction between nerves and brain is a complex system of electrical and chemical messages – some body parts such as the fingers, which are highly sensitive, will have greater representation than others.

PANIC ATTACKS

Anyone who has experienced a panic attack will tell you that they thought they were having a heart attack or were about to die. They really are incredibly frightening and occur suddenly for no apparent reason. Sometimes the panic attack is a reaction to a specific situation that has been causing concern, but often I see people who weren't aware they were feeling particularly anxious when the attack happened.

WHAT ARE THE SYMPTOMS?

Symptoms include palpitations (see p.61), sometimes accompanied by chest pain, lightheadedness or dizziness, a feeling that you can't take a proper breath, and tingling in your hands and fingers.

During a panic attack, your breathing is shallower and faster than usual, as a result you "blow off" more carbon dioxide than usual, which eventually affects the pH of your blood. And it is this change that causes the tingling feeling in your hands and fingers.

DEALING WITH PANIC ATTACKS

When a person is having a panic attack, he or she needs lots of calm reassurance. Try to get the person to breathe in and out of a paper bag; the bag must be paper (to avoid the possibility of suffocation) and the person must hold the bag so that it covers the mouth and nose. Using this method causes some of the exhaled carbon dioxide to be rebreathed back into the lungs. Eventually this raises carbon dioxide levels in the blood and the pH level returns to normal, although it may take several minutes to take effect and alleviate the symptoms.

DO PANIC ATTACKS NEED MEDICAL HELP?

An isolated attack is generally harmless and does not need medical help, but recurrent attacks could be a sign of an underlying anxiety problem or even depression and may require medication. Cognitive behavioural therapy teaches you how to recognize the early warning signs and control your attacks. It is often a time-consuming process but it works really well.

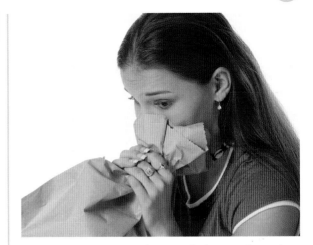

▲ *Rebreathing into a paper bag can alleviate symptoms of a panic attack.*

FIND OUT MORE
www.nopanic.org.uk

? DID YOU KNOW
Why you can't tickle yourself

When you stop to consider just how sophisticated and complex the human brain is, it's amazing that it doesn't go wrong more often. Have you ever wondered, for example, why you can tickle other people, but you can't tickle yourself?

The explanation lies in the fact that the cerebral cortex, the part of your brain that's responsible for the sensations of touch and pleasure (among other things), seems to fire more strongly in response to a stimulus from another person than from yourself, and most strongly when triggered by a stranger. Hence a tickle from someone you don't know may feel unpleasant, or even painful, but a tickle from a loved one can be fun and enjoyable.

According to Charles Darwin, tickling is a part of social bonding and, since we have no need to bond with ourselves, we can't trigger the mechanisms that result in ticklishness. It's an interesting theory and researchers have shown that gorillas and chimpanzees are ticklish too, which could lend support to it.

STRESS

It's impossible to lead a totally stress-free existence, and in fact you wouldn't want to. A little bit of stress makes you alert and helps you to get things done. Stress is also part of your "fight or flight" reflex and is a very important survival tool. Your ancestors, when faced with a mammoth, would find that their autonomic nervous system kicked in, causing a rise in adrenaline levels so that they could either stand and fight the mammoth or run away from it. Today, you may not come across any mammoths but an exam or an important job interview can trigger the same reaction and cause you to feel stressed.

GOOD AND BAD STRESS
Whether stress is positive or negative depends on the degree of stress. If, for example, when you go for an interview you are so stressed that you abuse the interview panel or run out of the room, you are hardly likely to get the job! But if you have just enough adrenaline running through your veins to make you mentally sharp, then stress is a positive thing.

Stress is also supposed to be short-lived, coming in bursts. As soon as the "mammoth" is out of sight, your adrenaline level starts to fall. Today, if your "mammoth"

is, for example, constant time pressure at work that never lets up, then you will be constantly firing on adrenaline and it's only a matter of time before it starts to take its toll on your health.

WHAT ARE THE PHYSICAL EFFECTS OF STRESS?
In the first, acute phase, stress causes your heart to beat faster, your blood pressure to rise, the pupils of your eyes to dilate, and your breathing to get faster. Blood is diverted away from the skin and internal organs towards the muscles and your blood sugar levels rise. All these things put us in a perfect position for the fight or flight response. If the situation is dealt with, then the body returns to normal. However, if it persists (as in constant time pressure), it can have a detrimental effect on your health – something has to give.

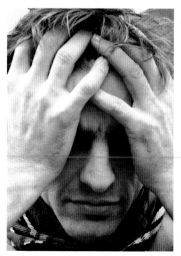

◄ Constant, long-term stress can adversely affect your health.

> ### DR DAWN'S HEALTH CHECK
> #### How to manage stress
> • Make a list of everything you have to do today. Then prioritize each task – if there are ten things on the list, the chances are you only need to do the first five and the rest can wait.
> • Delegate – you can't do everything for everyone and your kids may not load the dishwasher as well as you but they can certainly try.
> • Have the courage to say no. If you haven't got time to do something, say so. It is much better to be up front than to let people down at the last minute. There are only 24 hours in a day and, try as you might, you won't find any more (and some of those you need for sleep).
> • Find some "me time" – it doesn't matter if it's an evening with a friend or a session at a health spa. It helps you to switch off and you'll be more efficient the following day.
> • Take some exercise – even if it's just walking home. Regular exercise actually reduces stress levels.
> • Learn some relaxation techniques.
> • Accept offers of help, whether it's from a colleague in the office or another parent at the school gate. If someone is offering to do something for you, he or she can probably see that you are under pressure and wants to help.

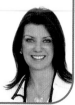

Putting aside time for yourself, with a professional massage for example, can be helpful in managing stress. ▶

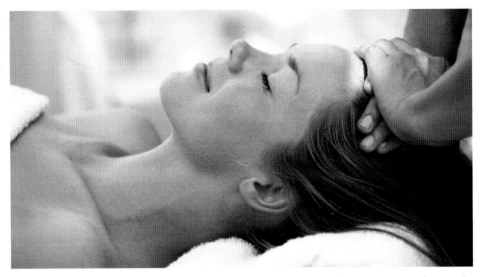

Illnesses that may be related to stress include:
- Depression (see p.180) and panic attacks (see p.177).
- Suffering from frequent minor infections because stress has weakened your immune system.
- Migraines (see p.184).

▾ Relaxation techniques, such as some yoga postures, can help reduce stress.

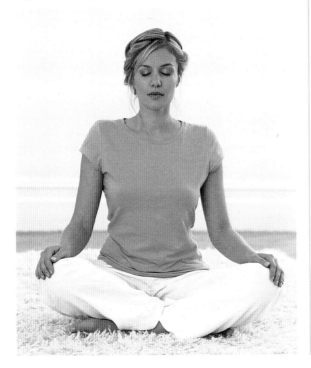

- Inflamed skin, such as a flare-up of eczema (see p.35) or psoriasis (see p.36).
- Indigestion (see p.85) and irritable bowel syndrome (see p.90).
- High blood pressure (see p.48), and even coronary heart disease (see p.52).

IS YOUR STRESS CONTROLLED?

So how do you know if you are too stressed? If you feel mentally alert, physically well, and can switch off at the end of the day, then you have your stress levels under control. But if, on the other hand, you are constantly anxious, find you are becoming less efficient because you are so swamped, or have physical symptoms related to stress, then you need to look at what is causing your stress and what you can do about it. For the sake of your health, you need to do this sooner rather than later.

TALK TO YOUR DOCTOR

Most of us can manage stress with a few simple adjustments to our lives but if you are struggling, your stress means you can't see your way through each day, or it's making you physically unwell, please talk to your doctor – he or she can help.

> **FIND OUT MORE**
> **www.bbc.co.uk/health**

DEPRESSION

This is the third most common reason for people to consult their doctor, and one in five of us will be affected by it at some point in our lives. Interestingly, only 20 per cent of those suffering from depression consult their doctor because of an emotional problem.

TIRED ALL THE TIME

Probably the most common manifestation of depression I see is patients coming into my surgery telling me that they feel "tired all the time". This is such a common problem that if you type "TATT" into any NHS computer, it will automatically come up with "tired all the time". Of course, there are lots of physical causes for feeling exhausted, such as anaemia, thyroid disease, and liver and kidney problems, to name but a few. I always run tests to rule these out; nine times out of ten the test results come back as normal and I end up talking to

▼ *Admitting that you are depressed and talking about it with somebody are important first steps to recovery.*

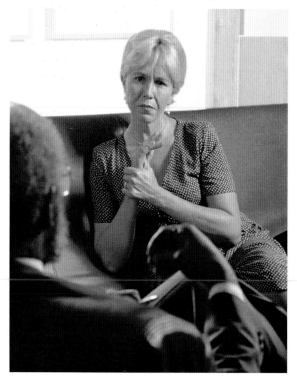

my patients about considering the effects of the stresses and strains of modern life, and the possibility that they could be depressed. Depression can, of course, be responsible for physical symptoms in its own right, including weight loss, early morning wakening, and loss of appetite, so the picture is not always clear.

DEPRESSION IS A PHYSICAL ILLNESS

Sadly, there is still stigma attached to mental illness. I often see patients who tell me they feel they should be able to "pull themselves together" or those who feel guilty about their depression. My answer to that is that depression is a physical illness – it is caused by an imbalance of chemicals in the brain. If it wasn't, antidepressant medication (which works by rebalancing those chemicals) would be useless, and it's not – it works extremely well for lots of people.

ANTIDEPRESSANTS CAN REALLY HELP

In fact, antidepressants work so well that many people are tempted to stop treatment after a couple of months because they feel so much better. If that is you, beware – if you start antidepressants, you should aim to stick with them for at least six months and maybe a year. It is a well-documented fact that if you stop them early you run the risk of a rebound. If you are thinking about stopping your antidepressants, talk to your doctor first. I usually suggest that people wean themselves off slowly, for example by taking their medication on alternate days for two or three weeks first. It's always a good idea to plan the timing too – if you are just about to go through the stress of a house move, now may not be the right time, or if you know that winter tends to make you more miserable even when you are not depressed, then why not wait until spring to reduce your treatment?

If you are not happy with the medication you are on, don't just stop it – talk to your doctor. There are so many different antidepressants available that he or she will almost certainly be able to find you a suitable alternative.

ARE ANTIDEPRESSANTS ADDICTIVE?

Many people worry about becoming "hooked" on antidepressants, but they are not addictive. Stopping them abruptly can cause withdrawal effects such as agitation, which may be confused with addiction, but it is quite different and weaning yourself off the medication slowly will avoid any problems with this.

ARE THERE ANY HERBAL REMEDIES FOR DEPRESSION?

There is one herbal remedy in particular – St John's wort – that, taken daily, is highly effective at treating mild to moderate depression and anxiety and is very popular with my patients.

A word of warning, though – herbal remedies are not as strictly regulated as conventional medicines, and like all things in this world, you get what you pay for. Cheapest is not necessarily best – I advise that you stick to a recognized brand. And always tell your doctor if you intend trying St John's wort as it can interfere with the action of some prescription and over-the-counter drugs, including the combined contraceptive pill.

CAN YOU TREAT DEPRESSION WITHOUT MEDICATION?

Yes, definitely! In fact, my first line with mild to moderate depression is to try other things first and these include:

Regular exercise can boost your energy levels and help combat depression. ▸

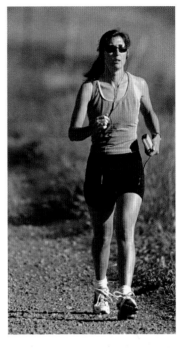

• Exercise – depression is associated with fatigue, lethargy, and lack of motivation, but if you can force yourself to take regular exercise, you will boost your energy levels, which can help you feel more positive. And this could start a virtuous cycle: the exercise makes you feel more positive and energetic, which means you are likely to exercise more, which makes you feel better, and so on.
• Massage – helps beat tension and promote relaxation.
• Cognitive behavioural therapy (CBT) – this is what I call one of the "talking therapies". It works by first teaching you how to recognize negative thoughts and the way they make you behave. Then it teaches you how to turn these thoughts around. CBT is highly effective but it is time-consuming and its availability on the NHS is limited. Work is being done in developing a computerized form of CBT called "Beating the Blues" – your doctor will know if it is available in your area.

DR DAWN'S HEALTH CHECK
Recognizing depression

Depression creeps up on you insidiously and it can be difficult to recognize. The symptoms to look out for include:
• Lack of motivation.
• Constant fatigue.
• Persistent negative thoughts and feelings of hopelessness.
• Poor sleep – particularly early morning wakening.
• Reduced appetite.
• No sex drive.
If you could be depressed, admitting it and talking about it are the first steps to getting better. Depression is nothing to be ashamed of, but unfortunately it is unlikely to simply go away if you ignore it, so please tell someone and do it today. The same applies if you think someone you know is depressed, talk to that person and encourage him or her to open up.

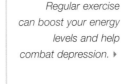

FIND OUT MORE
www.mind.org.uk

POSTNATAL DEPRESSION

It is normal to have the "baby blues" three or four days after a baby is born. This is the time when new mothers often become tearful and emotional. It is thought to be linked to the sudden fall in oestrogen levels after pregnancy, and is almost certainly made worse by exhaustion and sleep deprivation. But the baby blues is short-lived and it is quite different from postnatal depression.

HOW COMMON IS IT?

Postnatal depression is much more common than people think and it affects as many as one in ten women. It can occur any time within six months of the birth, and it's difficult to predict what form it will take and how severe it will be. Several antenatal treatments have been tried in a bid to prevent it, but without much success. However, health professionals are definitely better at recognizing postnatal depression and all new mothers are now asked by their health visitor to complete a questionnaire designed to flag up those at risk.

WHAT YOU CAN DO

If you think you might be suffering from postnatal depression, remember that you are not on your own – tell someone, preferably your health visitor and/or doctor, as they can help you. The following will also help:
• Make sure you eat and drink enough to allow for breastfeeding.
• Drink caffeine only in moderation – don't forget tea

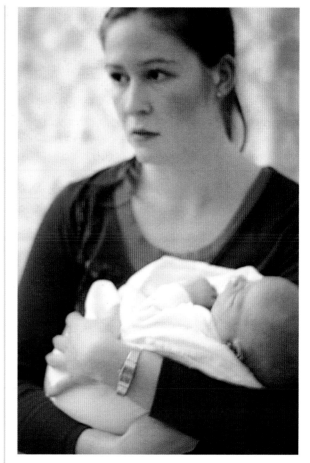

▲ *Postnatal depression affects up to one in ten women and may occur at any time in the six months after the birth.*

and cola drinks contain caffeine too.
• Don't smoke.
• Exercise moderately – take your baby for a walk, or arrange for your partner to look after the baby while you go out on your own.
• Rest whenever you can and certainly when you need to.
• Accept help with your baby when it is offered.

DR DAWN'S HEALTH CHECK
Recognizing postnatal depression

Common symptoms of postnatal depression include:
• Feeling tearful and overwhelmed a lot of the time.
• Difficulty bonding with your new baby.
• Being irritable – this may be with your baby but could also be with your partner or other children.
• Difficulty getting to sleep, even though you are very tired.
• Feeling hopeless as a mother.

FIND OUT MORE
www.apni.org.uk
www.mama.co.uk

CHRONIC FATIGUE SYNDROME

Some people suffer from a debilitating fatigue that lasts several months. It is usually triggered by an infection but less commonly by injury, stress, or even surgery. This is referred to as chronic fatigue syndrome (CFS) or ME. The diagnosis is often difficult because there are no specific tests or examination findings and people can have CFS for months before being diagnosed.

WHAT YOU CAN DO

The only treatments proven to help are graded exercise and cognitive behavioural therapy (CBT). For each, you will need a programme tailored to your symptoms. I find it useful to ask patients to keep a symptom and sleep diary for two weeks before they start any treatment regime.

You may find that your tiredness increases 24–48 hours after a period of exercise, and it's important to bear this in mind and increase your exercise levels very gradually. As harsh as it may sound, though, excessive rest should be avoided – research shows that it delays your recovery in the long run.

SEASONAL AFFECTIVE DISORDER

Everyone feels feel a bit low when the nights draw in and the weather becomes cold and miserable, but for over half a million people in this country the changing seasons herald more than just the "winter blues". Seasonal affective disorder (SAD) affects these people in varying degrees any time from September through to April, and in particular from December to February.

WHAT ARE THE SYMPTOMS?

During the autumn and winter months, people with this condition feel depressed, irritable, lethargic, and often have difficulty sleeping and reduced or no sex drive. Cravings for high-carbohydrate and sweet "comfort foods" are also common, and the inevitable weight gain from such a diet only compounds the low mood.

IS THERE ANY TREATMENT?

SAD is caused by a chemical imbalance in part of the brain called the hypothalamus, which is triggered by a lack of sunlight. If you have a mild form of SAD, just getting out into natural daylight for part of each day may be enough, but in more severe cases, light therapy may be required. This involves sitting in front of a special lightbox for anything from half an hour to four hours a day, depending on the intensity of light produced by the lightbox. You can read or write while sitting in front of the lightbox but you mustn't wear tinted glasses. You don't need to look directly at the light but if you do so, it will not damage your eyes. The results are astonishing – 85 per cent of sufferers notice an improvement, often in as little as a few days.

Unfortunately, the special lightboxes are only available privately, although some companies do offer a "try before you buy" scheme, and the Seasonal Affective Disorder Association (website below) has lightboxes for loan.

▼ Daily sessions in front of special lightboxes that produce very high-intensity light is effective for most SAD sufferers.

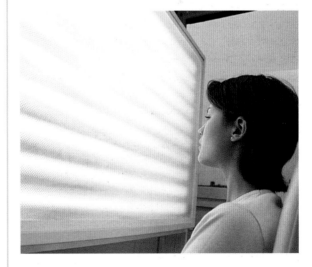

FIND OUT MORE
www.sada.org.uk

MIGRAINE

This is a condition that classically causes headache, visual disturbances, and nausea. It seems to be related to changes that take place in the blood vessels that supply the brain and scalp, but this certainly isn't the whole story. Migraine affects over six million people in the UK and two-thirds of them are women. Many sufferers have jobs and families, so the impact of migraine extends well beyond the sufferers themselves.

WHAT CAUSES IT?

The exact cause of migraine remains the subject of much debate. One thing we know for sure is that there are a lot of trigger factors – things that provoke an attack – such as stress, lack of food, smoking, hormone changes associated with a woman's periods, tiredness, foods such as chocolate and cheese, and drinks like coffee, tea, orange juice, and red wine. Identifying and avoiding trigger factors is an important part of managing migraine, but it can be surprisingly difficult, even for an experienced doctor.

I once worked with a migraine specialist who took months to realize that his own migraines always occurred on a Thursday. His Thursdays were long and hectic – he never had time to sit down and lived off coffee. Lunch was a bar of chocolate while on his way to the next packed clinic. The only rest he got was when he finally collapsed at home with a large glass of red wine. My

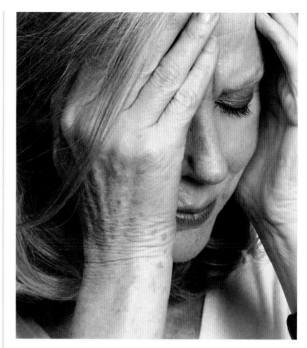

▲ *Migraine classically produces a headache, disturbances of vision, and nausea.*

colleague could hardly have had a fuller house of triggers to provoke a migraine attack.

WHAT YOU CAN DO

Keep a migraine diary. Write down everything you eat, when the migraine starts, its severity, and so on. This can

▼ *Chocolate is one of the common migraine triggers.*

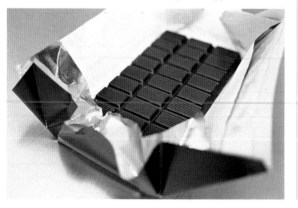

 DR DAWN'S HEALTH CHECK
Recognizing migraine

There are five stages of a migraine attack, although not all sufferers experience all stages.
1) Premonitory phase – may occur up to 24 hours before an attack and may include mood changes, fatigue, neck stiffness, and aversion to bright lights or noise.
2) Aura phase – about one in six sufferers experiences flashing lights, zig-zag vision, or blind spots.
3) Headache phase – usually one-sided; often with nausea/vomiting and sensitivity to light.
4) Resolution phase – often associated with a need for deep sleep.
5) Recovery phase – feeling "hung over" for anything up to 24 hours after an attack.

help you to identify the particular factors that trigger your migraines and simply avoiding those will go a long way to controlling your attacks.

Those who suffer the occasional migraine attack can usually cope with simple pain-relief tablets or prescription medication taken as soon as it starts. Anyone who suffers from weekly migraines should talk to their doctor. He or she can prescribe medication to prevent migraines.

WHAT ABOUT NON-DRUG TREATMENTS FOR MIGRAINE?

Many people are uncomfortable about taking long-term medication to control migraine and lots of alternative therapies have been tried. Below are listed some of the more common ones that my patients have found useful. There is no guarantee that they will work in your particular case, but you might find them worth trying if you are really averse to long-term medication.

- Acupuncture.
- Osteopathy.
- Relaxation therapy.
- Vitamin B2 – 400mg per day.

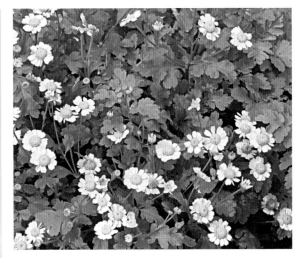

▲ *Feverfew leaves, fresh or dried, may help control migraine.*

- Magnesium – 500mg per day.
- Feverfew – a daily dose of 4–6 fresh leaves or 50mg in the dried form.
- Wearing a dental guard at night to stop you grinding your teeth.
- Botulinum toxin (botox) injections into the muscles around the skull have been known to help.

? DID YOU KNOW
Cluster headaches
More common in men, these headaches occur in bouts, often every day or night, for up to 12 weeks and then disappear. After one bout, most people have further attacks, often at the same time of the year. In the early stages, cluster headaches are often mistaken for migraine because they tend to be one-sided. They may last from about 15 minutes to three hours and, at their worst, may occur several times a day; they may also be accompanied by red, watery eyes, a runny or bunged-up nose, facial sweating, and droopy eyelids.

Keeping a symptom diary will help the diagnosis and may also identify any triggers. Common triggers include alcohol, hot environments, and strong smells. Avoiding triggers may prevent attacks. However, many cluster headaches occur without a pattern or obvious trigger and are therefore difficult to predict; if this is the case, talk to your doctor – there are many prescription medicines to treat the headache when it occurs.

! SEEK MEDICAL ADVICE NOW
If you any of the following apply:
- Stiff neck and fever.
- You cannot face bright lights.
- You are unusually drowsy.
- You have tender pulses in your temples.
- Your vision is disturbed.
- Your headache is worse in the morning, or when you cough, sneeze, or bend over.
- Your headache is getting progressively worse.
Most of us get headaches from time to time and they are nothing serious to worry about, although the very young and the very elderly don't tend to get headaches, so I would have a lower threshold for getting them checked out.

FIND OUT MORE
www.migraine.org.uk

EATING DISORDERS

Eating disorders start most frequently during adolescence. Our bodies are changing dramatically around this time and weight gain is an inevitable part of that. One in three adolescents starts dieting as a teenager. For most, it's a normal part of growing up, but for a minority it heralds the beginning of a morbid preoccupation with weight and body shape that could lead to an eating disorder.

HOW COMMON ARE EATING DISORDERS?

Anorexia nervosa is the third most common chronic illness of adolescence, affecting as many as one in 200 teenage girls, and bulimia is twice as common. The secretive nature of teenagers means that early signs are often missed. Anorexia is easier to spot than bulimia because of the weight loss, and girls may also stop their periods. Bulimics tend to be a normal weight and may go for years without being diagnosed.

ANOREXIA NERVOSA

Lots of teenage girls go on a diet to lose puppy fat, but in a few this dieting gets out of control and can lead to anorexia. Although it is less common in boys, about one in ten sufferers is male. Common features of anorexia include:

• Behavioural – anorexics are likely to become increasingly introverted and serious. They are often obsessed with food and lie about their eating habits. They may show other obsessions, including extreme tidiness or cleanliness. You may also notice a change

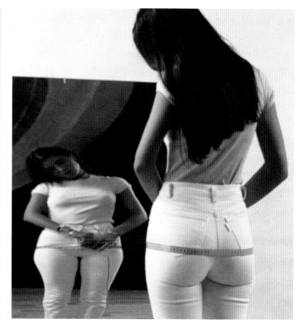
▲ Anorexics often have a distorted image of their body size.

in their style of dress – anorexics often choose baggy clothes to conceal their weight loss.
• Physical – apart from the obvious weight loss, anorexic girls often stop their periods if their weight falls below 44kg (7 stone). Boys and girls may have difficulty sleeping, feel constantly cold, and may complain of constipation, dizzy spells, and poor concentration.
• Emotional – anorexics have an intense fear of gaining weight. They have a distorted perception of their body size and shape, and often develop mood swings or become depressed.

BULIMIA

As many as four in ten women will develop some signs of bulimia in their lifetime. Common features include:
• Behavioural – bulimics often eat vast amounts of food in one sitting. You may also notice food wrappers in dustbins. Beware also the teenager who constantly disappears from the dinner table to the toilet – they may be going to vomit.
• Physical – most bulimics maintain a healthy weight, but physical signs to look out for include recurrent mouth infections and sore throats, sensitive or damaged teeth, bad breath, indigestion, and poor sleep patterns.

> **? DID YOU KNOW**
> **Who is at risk?**
> Anyone can suffer from an eating disorder, but those more at risk include:
> • Women – about 90 per cent of sufferers are female.
> • Those aged 15–25.
> • High-achieving perfectionist personalities.
> • Those with a middle-class background.
> • Those coming from a family with high expectations.
> • Those who have a relative with an eating disorder.

• Emotional – bulimics classically feel ashamed and guilty, which can manifest itself as mood swings.

WHAT TREATMENT IS AVAILABLE?

Accepting that you or a member of your family has an eating disorder is not easy, and tackling the problem is not about trying to force the person to eat. Treatment for eating disorders is longwinded and involves a team of doctors, nurses, and specialists. The more family support, the better the outcome.

Sadly, anorexia is, in effect, self-starvation and every year some anorexics succumb to their disease. There is also a high suicide rate among anorexics and an increased risk of drug or alcohol abuse. Bottom line? Never give up trying to help any member of your family who has an eating disorder.

DR DAWN'S HEALTH CHECK
Recognizing eating disorders

Telltale signs that could suggest that your son or daughter has an eating disorder include:

• Missing meals or eating alone – beware the teenager who has always "just eaten" somewhere else. He or she may be trying to conceal how little they are actually eating.

• A lack of concern or denial about weight loss – losing weight with no explanation usually worries people. If someone you know is not concerned by obvious weight loss, talk to them about it – if he or she denies being thin, this could be a warning sign.

• A sudden obsession with exercise without a specific goal like a marathon.

• Dental decay and burst blood vessels around the eyes can indicate that a person is forcing him- or herself to vomit.

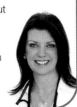

FIND OUT MORE
www.b-eat.co.uk

MEMORY LOSS

Most people will tell you that after cancer and heart disease, their biggest fear is memory loss and mental decline.

NORMAL MEMORY LOSS

It's completely normal to find that as you age your memory isn't as good as it used to be. I tell my patients to think of their brain as a suitcase – when we were young, the suitcase was relatively empty and everything you put in it stayed there. As you get older the suitcase gets fuller and fuller, until eventually when you put something in the front, something else has to fall out to make space. In fact, the analogy isn't perfect because when we start to lose our memory, it's the short-term memory that goes, but it makes the point. We may struggle to remember where we left our car keys or what time we were supposed to be at the dentist but we can remember the minute details of a family wedding 20 years ago.

WHEN IS IT NOT JUST FORGETFULNESS?

So how do you know whether you are just getting a bit forgetful, or if there is something more sinister about your memory loss? Let's go back to the car keys analogy – it's normal to forget where you put your car keys, we all do it from time to time, but what's not normal is to forget what you use them for. People with dementia (including Alzheimer's disease, the most common form of dementia) are persistently forgetful. They don't have the odd bad day and they get progressively worse over time.

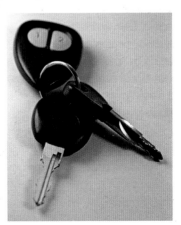

Occasional lapses of memory, such as forgetting where we put the car keys, are a normal part of ageing. ▶

Doctors use something called a mini-mental-state test to assess a person's memory. This consists of a series of questions that assess mental agility. The questions include things like asking what day, month, and year it is, remembering three objects, counting back from 100 in 7's (100, 93, 86, 79 …), and following a three-point command such as "take this piece of paper in your right hand, fold it in half, and then put it on the floor". The test has a maximum score of 30, and a score of less than 20 is highly suggestive of dementia.

ARE PREGNANT WOMEN MORE FORGETFUL?

Anecdotally, I would have to say yes! I have always been blessed with an excellent memory but during my first pregnancy I forgot to go to dinner parties and even struggled to remember where I had parked my car. I used to call it "mushy pea-brain of pregnancy" and it was so marked that by the time I was pregnant with our third child, we diagnosed the pregnancy on my not being able to remember our neighbour's phone number. Fortunately, though, memory comes back afterwards.

In fact, there is very little research into this and what exists is conflicting. Some studies claim that pregnant women have poorer memories, while others show no difference. Bottom line? It's a good excuse if you happen to forget an important birthday!

CAN YOU DO ANYTHING ABOUT MEMORY LOSS?

It seems that the memory is a bit like muscle – if you use it, it will get stronger, or at least won't deteriorate as quickly. So you can stave off the "normal" deterioration of memory that comes with age by keeping mentally active. Even simple things help, like doing crosswords, sudoku, or other puzzles and keeping up with current affairs by reading a newspaper. There is some evidence that regular exercise may help keep you mentally sharp; it certainly won't do any harm and will keep you physically fit, so give it a try.

ALZHEIMER'S DISEASE

This is the most common form of dementia, and accounts for around two-thirds of cases. Another common cause of dementia is vascular disease (strokes).

WHAT ARE THE SYMPTOMS?

In the early stages, Alzheimer's disease shows as loss of short-term memory but as it progresses, mental faculties progressively deteriorate. Sufferers neglect to look after themselves, become confused and aggressive, and may not even recognize their own families. It's a cruel disease, and most sufferers die within eight years of diagnosis.

CAN ALZHEIMER'S BE TREATED?

Sadly, all we can do is try to slow the progression of the disease. The measures in the box (right) will help. Reminiscing may keep the memory stimulated, and some patients find music therapy and aromatherapy useful. There are drugs that improve memory in Alzheimer's sufferers but they are restricted to those with moderate disease. If a family member suffers from Alzheimer's, ask their doctor if they'd be eligible for one of these drugs.

GINKGO BILOBA AND MEMORY

Ginkgo is thought to improve blood flow in the brain. It won't boost brain power in normal people but may slow deterioration in those with dementia. There is not yet enough research to say whether it definitely helps but may be worth a try.

? **DID YOU KNOW**
Who is at risk?

• People who have a relative with dementia – several genes have been identified that appear to play a role in developing Alzheimer's disease.
• People with high blood pressure.
• People with diabetes.
• Increasing age – one in 20 people over the age of 65 has a degree of dementia, but this rises to one in five over the age of 80.
• People who drink excessively.
• People with a history of head injury.

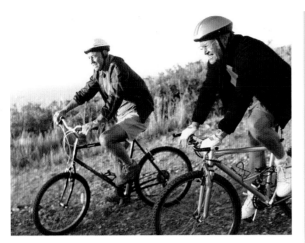

 Taking regular exercise will help reduce your risk of developing dementia.

DR DAWN'S HEALTH CHECK
Reducing your risk of dementia

There are some things you can do nothing about, such as increasing age or your family history, but there are some simple lifestyle measures worth adopting to minimize your risk of developing dementia:

• Don't smoke.
• Keep to the recommended alcohol limits.
• Get your blood pressure checked regularly, and have treatment if necessary.
• Keep your cholesterol levels within normal limits.
• Make sure you eat five portions of fruit and vegetables a day.
• Keep your saturated fat and salt intakes to a minimum.
• Eat oily fish every week.
• Take regular exercise.
• Protect your head – wear a helmet when you are cycling or riding a horse.
• Use your brain – it's like anything else: if you don't use it, you will lose it. So whether it's keeping up with current affairs or doing the crossword, keep your brain active and it will last longer.

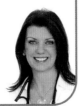

FIND OUT MORE
www.alzhelmers.org.uk

STROKE

Also known as a cerebrovascular accident (CVA), a stroke occurs when the blood flow to part of the brain is interrupted for more than a few minutes, which causes the affected part of the brain to be starved of oxygen and damaged, often permanently. Strokes are very common – every year in the UK 120,000 people have a first stroke and over 30,000 have a recurrent stroke.

WHAT ARE THE CAUSES?

A stroke can be caused by bleeding into the brain from a burst blood vessel or, more commonly, by blockage in one of the blood vessels. The resulting brain damage depends on the part of the brain affected. If the blood flow is only briefly impaired, then the person may suffer what's often called a "mini-stroke", or transient ischaemic attack (TIA), in which the damage is short-lived and returns to normal within 24 hours.

WHAT ARE THE SYMPTOMS?

The exact symptoms of a stroke depend on which part of the brain is affected – some will have weakness or loss of movement down one side, whereas others lose vision or have difficulty speaking. Some people complain of a sudden, severe headache. If you notice these signs in someone, you should get medical help straight away.

HOW IS A STROKE DIAGNOSED?

Most strokes are diagnosed on how the symptoms developed and the physical signs, such as loss of use of a limb. Anyone with sudden onset of weakness down

! EMERGENCY – DIAL 999

Call an ambulance if you suspect a stroke. If the person is still conscious, help him or her to lie down with head and shoulders raised and supported. Loosen any clothing that's restricting the breathing and reassure him or her while you wait for the ambulance. If the person is unconscious, carry out the first-aid procedure for unconsciousness (see p.240).

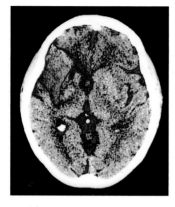

◄ *This brain scan of a stroke victim reveals a large area of brain damage (coloured orange).*

one side has had a stroke until proved otherwise. The important thing is to look for the cause. Eight out of ten strokes are due to a blockage, usually a blood clot, in an artery supplying the brain. The rest are caused by bleeding. They produce the same symptoms; the only way to tell the difference is with a CT scan. But it is important to differentiate between the two as the immediate treatment is different. A stroke caused by a blockage may respond to blood-thinning drugs, but if that treatment were given to someone whose stroke was caused by bleeding, the result could be catastrophic.

HOW RISKY IS A TIA?

Transient ischaemic attacks should be taken seriously – there is a one in ten chance of developing a full-blown stroke in the first week after a TIA. Taking something as simple as one aspirin a day could prevent that stroke so don't ignore the symptoms – consult your doctor.

HOW ARE STROKES TREATED?

Strokes caused by blood clots can respond well to blood-thinning agents called thrombolytics, but they should be given within three hours of developing symptoms. It is therefore vital that you get anyone who may have had a stroke to hospital as soon as possible.

WHAT IS THE LONG-TERM OUTLOOK?

Most of the recovery after a stroke occurs in the first three months, and intensive physiotherapy, occupational, and speech therapy helps rehabilitation. The full process may take up to about a year. Sadly, any disability left after a year is likely to be permanent, although a few patients do continue to improve afterwards.

DR DAWN'S HEALTH CHECK
Reducing your risk of further strokes

Unfortunately, about a third of those who have a stroke will die within a year, and those who survive are at increased risk of a further attack, so it's important that you minimize the risks, especially if you've had a stroke.

- If you smoke, give up.
- If you are overweight, lose the excess.
- Keep as active as possible.
- Prevent further clots. Eight out of ten strokes are caused by blood clots. If you have had a stroke your doctor will arrange a scan to confirm it. You will then be offered medication to help thin your blood and prevent further attacks. For some, this may simply mean taking an aspirin every day; for others, it will involve taking a drug called warfarin. This medication is unusual in that it doesn't have a standard dose – everyone reacts differently to it, and it doesn't necessarily depend on how big you are. Some people need 1mg on alternate days, while others may need 10mg every day to achieve the desired effect. This means that if you are taking warfarin you will need regular blood tests so that your doctor can fine-tune the dose to your specific requirements.
- Control your blood pressure. Taking medication to reduce blood pressure has been shown to reduce the risk of further strokes, even if your blood pressure wasn't high in the first place. If you have had a stroke, you will be put on medication to lower your blood pressure as soon as the initial healing process is established – usually within a few days or weeks.
- Lower your cholesterol. If your stroke was caused by a blood clot, your doctor will advise you to take medication to reduce your cholesterol levels – again, even if your levels were normal in the first place. The theory behind this is that whatever your cholesterol level was, it was enough for you to have furred-up arteries and it should be lower.

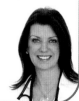

FIND OUT MORE
www.stroke.org.uk

EPILEPSY

Epilepsy is the tendency to have recurrent seizures or fits, which are caused by a sudden burst of electrical activity in the brain that disrupts normal brain activity. The physical manifestations depend on where in the brain the electrical changes occur. There are around 40 different types of seizure, ranging from momentary absences to full-blown fits with unconsciousness and uncontrollable jerking of the limbs.

WHAT CAUSES EPILEPSY?
Sometimes epilepsy is caused by damage to the brain – from oxygen starvation at birth, a head injury, meningitis, or even following a stroke; but in around six out of ten cases we simply don't know why it happens.

HOW IS EPILEPSY DIAGNOSED?
Most epileptics cannot recall their attacks' so if any friends or family have seen an attack, take them with you to your doctor to give an eyewitness account. If your doctor thinks it could be epilepsy, he will refer you to a specialist for tests, including an electroencephalogram (EEG) to measure the electrical activity of your brain.

WILL I HAVE TO TAKE MEDICATION FOR LIFE?
Anti-epileptic drugs control seizures but don't cure epilepsy. Some people who have been seizure-free for years may choose to try stopping the drugs. This must be done gradually and under close supervision by your doctor because of the risk that the fits will return.

WHAT ABOUT DRIVING WITH EPILEPSY?
If you have had a seizure, you must inform the DVLA. If you are diagnosed with epilepsy, you will be allowed to drive again when you have been fit-free for a year or have only had fits in your sleep for at least three years.

FIND OUT MORE
www.epilepsynse.org.uk

PARKINSON'S DISEASE

Parkinson's disease is a progressive degenerative disease of the brain that affects about 120,000 people in the UK, mainly those over 50.

WHAT ARE THE SYMPTOMS?
There are three main symptoms:
- Tremor – many sufferers develop a hand tremor that is noticeable at rest but goes when the hands are used.
- Stiffness – classic symptoms include difficulty getting up from a chair or turning over in bed, and some find that their face becomes stiff, resulting in a lack of expression.
- Slowness – called bradykinesia, this is a common problem in which initiating movements is difficult.

HOW IS PARKINSON'S TREATED?
Sadly there is no cure. Parkinson's patients have reduced levels of a brain chemical called dopamine and they need to take regular medication to replace or mimic the action of dopamine. This can mean taking several different drugs at frequent intervals to maintain mobility.

People with Parkinson's must inform the DVLA. You won't automatically be banned from driving but you may be asked to have a medical or do a driving test.

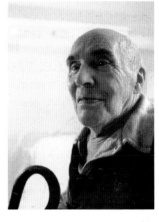

Some people with Parkinson's disease develop a stiff, expressionless face. ▶

FIND OUT MORE
www.parkinsons.org.uk

• Sleeping for at least 4 to 7 hours a night helps you to live longer • We produce growth hormones when we sleep – chronic sleep deprivation in developing children could mean they miss their full potential adult height by an inch or two • Being awake continuously for more than 18 hours could have a worse effect on your reaction times than having a blood alcohol level over the legal limit for driving • If we sleep for 8 hours we only spend one hour of it in our deepest sleep • Most dreams occur in the last third of our sleep time.

17

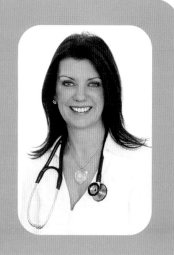

Sleep

Introduction When we sleep and when we wake is regulated by the brain and is influenced by external factors such as light and noise, and internal factors – chemicals and hormones like melatonin which is highest during sleep. The hours we spend asleep can be divided into two categories described by scientists as "REM" and "non-REM" sleep. REM stands for rapid eye movement and the distinction between the two types of sleep can be seen on a tracing of the electrical activity of the brain called an EEG (electroencephalogram).

Humans alternate between REM and non-REM sleep every 90 minutes. Non-REM sleep accounts for 75–80 per cent of total sleep time. It has four stages, each one being a deeper sleep than the one before. Interestingly, stage 4 non-REM sleep (the deepest sleep) predominates in the first third of the night, so there is some truth in the old wives tale that an hours sleep before midnight is worth two after.

How much sleep we need certainly varies from person to person, but as a rough guide, children under five years of age should be sleeping 11–13 hours a night whilst older kids (8–12) may need only 8–10 hours. It is generally accepted that 6–8 hours' sleep is optimum for most adults.

SNORING

Over three and half million people in the UK snore and most of them are men. When you sleep, the muscles in your throat relax along with the rest of you. The noise of snoring results from the vibration of the soft tissues of the airways as we breathe in and out.

WHAT YOU CAN DO

Being overweight, smoking, and drinking too much alcohol can make snoring worse, so a few lifestyle changes may help. You are also more likely to snore when you sleep on your back – one exasperated patient of mine cured her husband's snoring by sewing a tennis ball into the back of a nightshirt so that every time he rolled on to his back it was so uncomfortable that he rolled back again on to his side!

If you snore when you have a blocked nose, it may be worth trying a nasal spray, or nasal strips that help keep your nasal passages open. You can get these from your chemist.

HOUSE DUST ALLERGY

Allergy to the house dust mite is to blame in some cases and while you can never eradicate the mites completely, you can reduce their numbers by washing bedding, rugs, and curtains regularly and swapping feather pillows and duvets for non-allergenic synthetic bedding. Any soft toys should also be washed weekly and placed in a bag in the freezer for a day to kill the mites.

▼ *Sleeping on your back makes snoring more likely.*

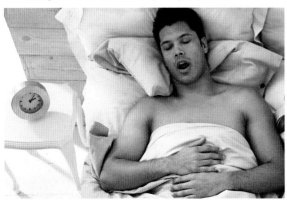

OBSTRUCTIVE SLEEP APNOEA

This is a condition in which you stop breathing for short periods of time while you are asleep. Obstructive sleep apnoea has become widely recognized as a problem only in the last 20 years or so. Each episode begins with a loud snoring or snorting noise, which is followed by a period of no breathing that can last up to 40 seconds, then you start to breathe again, often with a jolt. This can happen up to 400 times a night.

DIAGNOSIS AND TREATMENT

It is important that sleep apnoea is treated as, aside from the obvious risks associated with long-term sleep deprivation and daytime sleepiness, it carries an increased risk of high blood pressure (see p.49) and coronary heart disease (see p.52).

The diagnosis can generally be made from the story you tell your doctor, but it will be confirmed after observation in a sleep laboratory. The first line of treatment is to address the risk factors listed below. If these aren't enough, you will be given a device to wear at night called a CPAP (continuous positive airways pressure) machine, which feeds pressurized air into your airways to keep them open all night.

> **?** **DID YOU KNOW**
> **Who is at risk?**
> • Men are four times more likely to have sleep apnoea than women.
> • People who are overweight – excess fat around the neck especially makes it more likely for the airways to be squashed.
> • People who drink a lot of alcohol – alcohol is a relaxant and makes the muscles in the throat more relaxed.
> • Smokers – it's thought that tobacco smoke causes inflammation of the lining of the throat.
> • People who have a first-degree relative (parent, sibling, or child) with the condition.
> • People who are taking sedative drugs, such as sleeping tablets and diazepam.

INSOMNIA

Insomnia is the term we use to describe difficulty sleeping. There isn't a specific number of hours sleep below which I'd say someone is suffering from insomnia. Put simply, an insomniac is somebody who is consistently awake when they want to be asleep.

HOW MUCH SLEEP DO WE NEED?

How much sleep a person needs varies tremendously – you have all heard how Margaret Thatcher survived on just three hours a night during her leadership and at the other extreme there are people who claim not to be able to function on fewer than ten hours a night. It seems to me that between six and eight hours' sleep a night is the optimum for an adult. In fact, according to research from America, people who regularly get this amount of sleep actually live longer.

But of course, there is more to sleeping than the number of hours you spend in bed – the quality of sleep is just as important. A new mother may physically spend eight hours in bed, but if her sleep is constantly interrupted by her baby she won't get what I call good battery-recharging sleep.

Problems with sleeping are extremely common – all of us have the occasional night when we are worried about the next day and then toss and turn until the alarm goes off, but one in seven people has sleeping problems on a regular basis.

WHAT CAUSES INSOMNIA?

Common causes of insomnia include:
- Stress.
- Anger – there's nothing like a row late at night to ensure you won't sleep.
- Depression – people with depression may get off to sleep but they often wake in the early hours and then can't get back to sleep.
- Pain – this can often seem even worse at night.
- Noise – a partner who snores loudly is almost bound to disturb you.
- Room temperature – being too hot or too cold will adversely affect sleep.

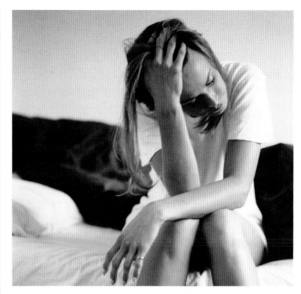

▲ *Long-term insomnia can be physically and mentally debilitating.*

- Medical problems, including thyroid disease, bladder problems, or prostate disease, that necessitate getting up for a wee at night.
- Caffeine – it is in coffee, tea, and cola.
- Alcohol – it interferes with natural sleep patterns.
- Nicotine – it raises the heart rate, blood pressure, and increases the levels of adrenaline .
- Drugs – some prescribed medicines can affect your sleep; talk to your doctor if you think this may be the cause of your insomnia.
- Jetlag (see p.205).

CAN SLEEPING TABLETS HELP?

Many people faced with several consecutive nights of poor sleep may well be tempted to resort to sleeping tablets. They will almost certainly work in the short term but they are certainly not a panacea, not least because they are highly addictive – taking them for as little as two weeks could have you hooked. This is one reason why your doctor may be reluctant to prescribe them.

WHAT ABOUT HERBAL REMEDIES?

The herbal remedy valerian has been used for centuries and does seem to help. Passion flower may also be worth a try, and lots of people report that a drop of lavender oil on the pillow improves their sleep pattern.

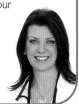
SLEEPWALKING

Sleepwalking is surprisingly common: almost half the population will sleepwalk at some time in their lives, mostly in childhood. If sleepwalking starts out of the blue as an adult, it is often linked to stress. The strange thing about sleepwalking is that you usually have no recollection of doing it. I have known people get up and make themselves a sandwich in their sleep but deny all knowledge in the morning! This is because, unlike dreaming, sleepwalking occurs in our deepest sleep.

TYPES OF SLEEP

During the night everyone oscillates between two types of sleep, which doctors describe as rapid eye movement (REM) sleep and non-rapid eye movement (NREM) sleep. You spend about a quarter of the night in REM sleep and the rest in NREM. You dream during REM sleep and if you are woken during REM sleep, you can often remember some of your dream. Sleepwalking, on the other hand, occurs during the deeper stages of NREM sleep, and it's normal to have no memory of activity during this sleep.

IS SLEEPWALKING SERIOUS?

Sleepwalking is only a problem if we fall over things or wander outside the house. If you sleepwalk regularly, it's worth arranging furniture to minimize the risk of injury and possibly even getting a stair gate for the top of the stairs to stop you falling down them.

IS IT DANGEROUS TO WAKE SOMEONE UP WHILE THEY ARE SLEEPWALKING?

Because sleepwalking occurs in your deepest sleep, if you wake someone abruptly from that state, he or she is likely to be disorientated and possibly distressed but nothing worse. But in fact there is no need to wake a sleepwalker, just quietly guide him or her back to bed.

- Always keep a sunscreen with you and reapply it regularly
- Be vigilant about the safety of food and water • Remember to pack insect repellents, safety nets, and medications if necessary • Take care with contraception when you are away – one in six British holiday makers under 30 has sex with a new partner on holiday, and half don't use a condom • Never underestimate the power of the sea and be careful about swimming in "fresh" water that could be laden with disease • Always put your personal safety first • Make sure that you have travel insurance when you go away, and carry the insurance company's telephone number with you.

18

Holiday & travel health

Introduction The world really has become a smaller place. It is estimated that 80 million people will travel from a developed country to a developing one every year, and across the globe 600 million people will travel abroad. When I was a junior doctor it was unusual to see tropical diseases in the UK, but in a short space of time the picture has totally changed.

As a doctor, I regularly receive information bulletins from the Department of Health advising on how UK doctors should manage suspected cases of anything from SARS to bird flu. Thankfully, serious illnesses contracted on holiday are still rare but spending your hard-earned holiday locked up in a hotel room feeling under the weather is not a good way to spend time. We have all heard horror stories of holidays being ruined by illness. Some sadly can't be avoided but some certainly can, and this chapter will give you a few tips to enable you and your family to keep the risk of being unwell while away to a minimum.

BEFORE YOU GO

If you plan ahead, your will enjoy you holiday far more. Before you go, find out whether you need vaccinations, get travel insurance, and make sure you have enough of any prescription medicines you need.

TRAVEL VACCINES

It is always best to think well ahead, particularly if you are planning a holiday somewhere exotic, as you will need vaccinations. You can go to a travel centre, or they can be given by the practice nurse at your doctor's surgery – for a fee. Some vaccines, like yellow fever, can only be given at certain approved centres. Which vaccinations you need will depend on where you are going and what vaccinations you have had in the past. Make an appointment to see the practice nurse at least eight weeks before you travel so that you have time to fit in all the vaccines – they can't all be given together and some need to be given more than once.

MEDICINES

If you are taking prescription medicines, make sure you have enough to last the holiday and some extra in case of delays. Make a note of the medical names and dosage (or take a copy of your prescription) so that, if you lose your medicines, you will be able get a local doctor to prescribe more. All drugs have two names, a generic name and a brand name, so write them both down. Carry your medicines in your hand luggage in case your hold luggage is delayed or lost or your flight is delayed; this is especially important if you have diabetes, or if you are on a long-haul flight. If you need to take needles and syringes with you, ask your doctor for a covering letter as airlines are, understandably, strict on what you are allowed in hand luggage.

As well as any prescription medicines, it's also worth taking a basic first-aid kit. Suggested contents of such a kit are shown on the right.

FITNESS TO FLY

If you have a medical condition that may affect your fitness to fly, check with your airline well in advance as there may be restrictions. For example, there may be a minimum time delay before you can fly after surgery, or you may not be allowed to fly beyond a certain number of weeks into pregnancy.

TRAVEL INSURANCE

Don't leave the country without travel insurance – the cost of treating even minor ailments in foreign countries can come as a nasty shock. Even more so if you need to be flown home! The UK has a reciprocal arrangement with many European countries, but you will need a European Health Insurance Card. You can apply for this on a form available from your post office or you can apply online at the website below.

> **! HOLIDAY FIRST AID KIT**
> **Along with any prescription medicines, your travel medicines should include:**
> - Paracetamol.
> - Anti-inflammatory medication such as ibuprofen.
> - Antihistamine creams and medication.
> - Antiseptic wipes and cream.
> - Insect repellent.
> - Travel sickness pills.
> - Diarrhoea medicine and rehydration salts.
> - Probiotic supplements.
> - Plasters, wound dressings, and maybe a bandage.
> - Sunscreen.

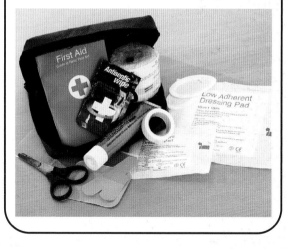

FIND OUT MORE
www.ehic.org.uk

TRAVEL SICKNESS

Many people suffer from travel sickness at some point, and it is particularly common in children. Luckily, there are various things you can do to prevent or minimize it.

WHAT YOU CAN DO

If you know that you are prone to travel sickness, eat only small amounts and don't drink alcohol before travelling. If you are flying, ask for a window seat near the wings of the plane as this is the most stable part of the aircraft and less likely to give you motion sickness. If you are travelling by ship, again try to sit in the middle of the ship, where you will experience the least motion. And if you are travelling by car, you will find sitting in the front seat is better than sitting in the back. While on the move, watch the horizon and don't try to read.

OTHER TREATMENTS

There are also various over-the-counter travel sickness medicines, which many people find effective. They should generally be taken before travelling. But beware, some of these medicines cause drowsiness and should therefore not be used if you are driving, and many also increase the effects of alcohol.

Some people find acupressure wristbands or natural remedies based on ginger are effective. They are certainly worth trying if the other remedies have failed or you don't want to use medication.

▾ *Acupressure wristbands may help prevent travel sickness.*

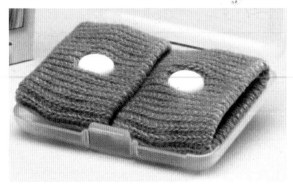

TRAVELLER'S DIARRHOEA

Diarrhoea can ruin your holiday, but you can minimize the risk of getting it by drinking only bottled water; washing any fruit or vegetables in bottled water; avoiding eating from street stalls; and being scrupulous about handwashing. You should use bottled water when brushing your teeth also.

HOW YOU CAN TREAT IT

If you do get a bout of diarrhoea, drink plenty of fluids to prevent dehydration – flat cola or lemonade is a good source of sugar if you are off food. You shouldn't take antidiarrhoea medication for the first couple of days – if you have a bug, it's better out of your body. After 48 hours most of the infection will have cleared from your body, but the diarrhoea may persist because you will have lost a lot of the good bacteria that live in your gut. It is safe at this point to take medication to stop the diarrhoea and it's also a good idea to top up your good bacteria with a probiotic. The diarrhoea should clear up completely within a week or so.

▾ *Drinking only bottled water can help prevent traveller's diarrhoea while on holiday.*

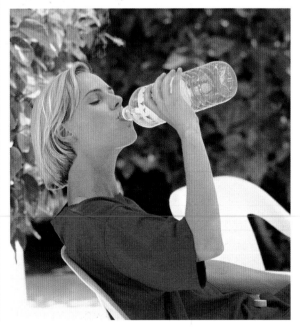

WHEN SHOULD YOU SEEK MEDICAL HELP?

You should see a doctor if:

- Your symptoms last more than a few days.
- You have severe abdominal pain.
- You notice blood or pus in the diarrhoea.

WHAT ABOUT ANTIBIOTICS?

Doctors don't generally prescribe antibiotics because most diarrhoeal illnesses are self-limiting, many are due to viruses (which don't respond to antibiotics), and most antibiotics can cause diarrhoea! The exception is for diarrhoea caught in developing countries, which is more frequently bacterial. In this instance, oral antibiotics can reduce the duration of the illness. If you are travelling to a high-risk area and will find it difficult to see a doctor, your own doctor may be willing to prescribe an antibiotic for you just in case.

PRICKLY HEAT

This is an itchy rash that can develop within hours of exposure to the sun but more commonly starts to form about three days after exposure. The most common sites are the chest, armpits, hands, and feet. The classic pink spots usually last for several days, and as well as being itchy may also produce a burning or prickling sensation. Unfortunately, if you or your children have suffered from prickly heat once, then the chances are that it will strike again.

WHAT CAUSES IT?

The problem seems to be due to an allergic reaction to sunlight, and in particular to UVA rays. These are the longer-wavelength rays in sunlight and they can pass through light clothing, glass, and clouds. And you don't have to be sitting on a baking hot beach to get prickly heat; you can get it when you are skiing, for example, because the sun is reflected off the snow.

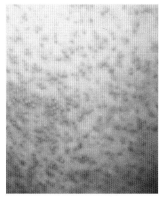

The characteristic raised, itchy, pink spots of prickly heat. ▶

WHAT YOU CAN DO

If you or your children suffer from prickly heat, try my tips in the box below. If prickly heat develops then stay out of the sun until the symptoms have cleared up. Calamine lotion will soothe, and steroid creams can also help. Antihistamines may reduce the itching but be careful – a side effect of some antihistamines is to make the skin more sensitive to the sun.

DR DAWN'S HEALTH CHECK
Reducing the chances of prickly heat

Prevention is better than cure – if your family have suffered in the past:

- Avoid the sun between 11am and 3pm when it is at its hottest.
- Restrict exposure to the sun and increase it gradually.
- Use sunscreen that has a high sun-protection factor (SPF) and a star-rating of three or four. SPF indicates the protection against UVB rays, and the star-rating indicates protection from UVA rays. Using a sunscreen without these may give you a false sense of security and actually make things worse!
- If you are not sure how strong the sun is, look at your shadow – if it is shorter than you, then the sun is strong and you need to protect yourself.

? DID YOU KNOW
Dr Dawn's beach tip

Rub talcum powder on to wet, sandy skin and all the grains of sand disappear like magic, making it easier to apply sunscreen to children on the beach.

HEAT EXHAUSTION AND HEATSTROKE

You should always drink eight to ten glasses of fluid a day (preferably water) but when the weather is very hot, you may need a lot more and it is easy to become dehydrated. The aim is not to let yourself get thirsty – some experts believe that by the time you feel thirsty, you are already slightly dehydrated.

HEAT EXHAUSTION

The symptoms of heat exhaustion include sweating (often with pale, clammy skin), headache, nausea, vomiting, and dizziness. If you start to experience these symptoms, you need to get out of the heat straight away (ideally into an air-conditioned building), drink plenty of cold fluids, remove excess clothing, and sponge yourself down with tepid (not cold) water.

HEATSTROKE

If the symptoms of heat exhaustion are ignored, they can develop into heatstroke, which can be fatal. The body's temperature control mechanisms fail and it becomes unable to lose heat. Instead of sweating, your skin becomes hot, red, and dry. If heatstroke develops, a person can rapidly become confused and disorientated and may lose consciousness. Heatstroke is a medical emergency that needs urgent attention in hospital (see box below).

> **! EMERGENCY – GET MEDICAL HELP**
> **Call an ambulance if a person has the following signs:**
> - Hot, dry skin.
> - A sudden headache.
> - A body temperature over 40°C (104°F).
> - He or she becomes confused and gradually loses consciousness.
>
> In the meantime, get the person out of the heat. Sponge the person with cold or tepid water, and fan the person to keep him or her cool.

SWIMMER'S EAR

Frequent exposure to water moistens the skin in the ear canal, which creates an ideal environment for bacteria and fungi to grow, a condition that is commonly referred to as "swimmer's ear".

HOW CAN I PREVENT IT?

If you are plagued with ear infections every time you go away, try using acid-alcohol ear drops, which are available over the counter from your chemist. Put three or four drops into your ear every day after swimming. Lie on your side to put them in and gently massage the area in front of your ear for a minute or two. Then turn over to your other side and repeat the process for the other ear. Wearing ear plugs while swimming also helps, but don't be tempted to push them deep into the ear and they should only be relied upon for surface swimming.

IS THERE ANY OTHER TREATMENT?

If you get swimmer's ear despite trying the measures above, you will probably need prescription ear drops containing antibiotics and/or steroids, which will need to be used several times a day for at least a week. During this time, you should avoid swimming and keep the ears dry with a shower cap or cotton wool plug coated in petroleum jelly when taking a shower or bath. If the condition is causing pain, using an over-the-counter painkiller such as paracetamol will help.

▾ *Swimmer's ear occurs when the ear canal is persistently moist and becomes infected.*

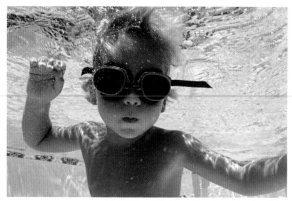

JETLAG

This occurs when travelling through time zones disrupts your body clock. It is worse when you travel from west to east. Time differences of five hours or fewer don't usually cause much problem, but greater than this and you suffer from fatigue, disorientation, and an inability to sleep.

WHAT CAUSES IT?

Your body clock is primed to respond to a regular rhythm of daylight and darkness, so it is "thrown" when it experiences daylight at what it considers the wrong time. It can take several days for the body clock to readjust to the new times, but by controlling your body's exposure to daylight you can trick your brain into beating jetlag more quickly.

WHAT ABOUT MELATONIN?

Melatonin is a hormone secreted at night by a gland in the brain called the pineal gland. It is thought to play a role in setting your normal sleep patterns. Pilots and cabin crew who regularly fly through time zones have used melatonin for years in an attempt to combat jetlag. Many swear by it but scientific studies have failed to prove any benefit and until its safety has been fully assessed, my advice would be to stick to the tips below.

DR DAWN'S HEALTH CHECK
If you are planning a long-haul flight:

• Set your watch to the time at your destination as soon as you board the plane.

• Try to eat and sleep according to appropriate times in your destination.

• Shut the window blind when it would be night-time in your destination.

• As soon as you arrive at your destination, spend some time outside in the daylight.

• Schedule any outings or commitments for times when your energy levels will be highest – in the evenings after flying east and in the mornings after flying west.

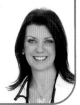

BLOOD CLOTS

Most people are aware that long-haul air travel can put you at risk of deep vein thrombosis (DVT, see p.60). The danger of this condition is that a blood clot that forms in your leg might break off and block a major blood vessel, causing what is called a pulmonary embolism, which can be fatal. Thankfully, this is rare and there are measures you can take to reduce the risk.

MINIMIZING YOUR RISK

If you think you might be at risk of a blood clot – perhaps because you have a family history of DVT, are taking the contraceptive pill or HRT, or have severe varicose veins – talk to your doctor before travelling. He or she will be able to advise whether it would be appropriate for you to take aspirin to thin the blood. If so, your doctor will probably recommend that you take aspirin the day before travel and on the day of departure.

During the flight, walk up and down every hour. When sitting, draw circles in the air with your feet to keep the blood circulating. Drink plenty of fluids but avoid caffeine and alcohol as these can dehydrate you. You can also buy antithrombus stockings (sometimes called just "flight socks") to wear during the flight.

▼ *Antithrombus stockings ("flight socks") worn during a long-haul flight may reduce the risk of a blood clot.*

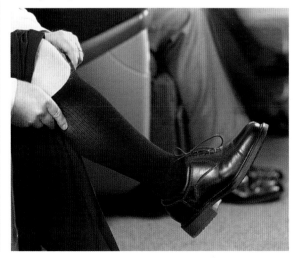

• As a rough guide, you can predict the adult height of your child by doubling the height at 18 months old for a girl or two years for a boy • During puberty, girls may grow 8cm (20in) in one year, while boys can grow an incredible 12cm (30 in) in the same time • It is possible to tell the difference between male and female babies at the 12th week of pregnancy • One in five boys and one in four girls of school age are clinically overweight • School children should exercise for one hour every day – at least half don't achieve this • Boys' and girls' brains really are different – even pre-school a girl is likely to be two months ahead of her male peers in speech, but the boys will have better spatial awareness.

19
Children's health

Introduction From the moment they are born (and probably before), our children are our most treasured posession, but they don't come with an instruction manual, and they have a nasty habit of going "wrong"! It doesn't matter how well qualified and in control you are in your life, as a parent you will be constantly questioning yourself and anxious as to whether you have done the right thing. Add to that the other trait of any parent – guilt – and it's easy to see why so many of us get stressed.

It is important to remember that there is help out there, and it's OK to ask for it. Trust your instincts. However insecure you may feel, you know your children better than anyone else, and if they are "not right" then ask for help. I am often asked for advice on sleeping, feeding, and behaviour. Sometimes all that is needed is some reassurance as to what is normal, sometimes the difficulties are better dealt with by a health visitor, and sometimes there is a medical problem that needs further attention. It is always better to ask than to sit at home and worry.

MANAGING A FEVER

Body temperature is normally around 37°C (98.6°F), but for some children it may be slightly higher or lower. A body temperature above this indicates fever, usually caused by infection, and it's the body's way of fighting illness. A slight rise won't hurt your child, but a temperature of over 40°C (104°F) can be serious as it can trigger febrile seizures in young children.

WHAT ARE THE SYMPTOMS?

As your child is developing a fever, he or she will shiver and if your child is old enough, they may complain of feeling cold. As the body temperature rises, your child will develop hot, flushed skin; he or she may also be sweating, and may complain of a headache.

WHAT YOU SHOULD DO

It is particularly important to control fever in young children. When your child has a fever, your natural instinct as a parent may be to wrap him or her up warm, but don't! As tough as it may sound, it is important to keep your child's temperature down at this point – strip him or her down to underwear, open the windows, and make sure your child has plenty of cold drinks. Give your child the recommended dose of liquid paracetamol or ibuprofen. Never give a child under 16 any medication

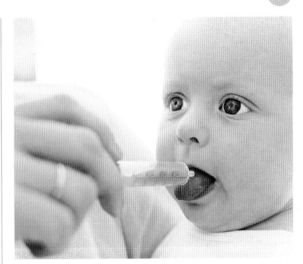

▲ *Children's liquid paracetamol or ibuprofen can help to manage a fever.*

containing aspirin. It can trigger a very rare condition called Reye's syndrome.

FEBRILE SEIZURES

If a fever is not controlled, one in 20 children between the ages of six months and six years will have a fit, or seizure, associated with it known as a febrile convulsion. These fits seem to be triggered by a rapid rise in temperature and they can be terrifying to witness. Classically, a child loses consciousness and becomes rigid, often jerking his or her limbs. After a few minutes, the child goes pale or even blue and limp, and may sleep very deeply. Children who have had one febrile seizure are more likely to have another one if they are ill again.

If your child does have a seizure, cool him or her as above. Protect them by putting soft padding around him or her. When the seizure stops, place your child on his or her side in the recovery position (see p.241), and call for medical advice.

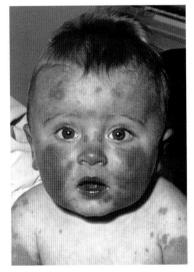

◄ *Infections such as parvovirus (slapped cheek disease) are a common cause of fever.*

> **! SEEK MEDICAL ADVICE NOW**
> **If your child:**
> • Has a temperature over 39°C (102.2°F).
> • Has a raised temperature accompanied by drowsiness.
> • Has a raised temperature with a febrile seizure (see above).

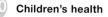
COUGHS AND COLDS

All children will get coughs and colds, and most are caused by a viral infection – in other words, antibiotics will not help. You have to supply tender loving care together with regular doses of children's liquid paracetamol or ibuprofen.

WHAT YOU CAN DO

Although chemists' shelves are full of cough remedies for every type of cough, most coughs will improve within a few days, so the virus should be allowed to run its course. Most will get better without any treatment, but see your doctor if a cough does not get better after three to four days. There is a small chance that your child could develop a secondary infection, such as pneumonia or bronchitis, while his or her immune system is low.

CROUP

Croup is a short, barking, dry cough that is a result of air breathed in through an inflamed windpipe. It is normally more noticeable at night, and your child will have difficulty breathing, especially inhaling. (It's distinct from asthma, which makes breathing out especially difficult, see p.65.) A dry, croupy cough often responds to steam – simply boiling a kettle in the room or putting hot, wet tea towels on any radiators will help. Alternatively, take your child into the bathroom, shut the doors and windows, and run the hot tap into the bath.

If your child's attack of croup is particularly severe, especially if he or she is having difficulty breathing, then you should seek medical advice immediately.

> **! SEEK MEDICAL ADVICE NOW**
> **If your child:**
> - Develops a high temperature.
> - Cannot sleep because of the cough.
> - Becomes short of breath.
> - Starts to develop a blue tinge to the skin.
> - Becomes floppy and lifeless.
> - Has a cough that does not improve after three to four days.

STICKY EYE

Some babies are born with blocked tear ducts that can take several months to open. This can cause a build-up of the natural secretions that normally drain through the ducts and it may look as if your baby has an eye infection.

DOES IT NEED TREATMENT?

Sticky eye rarely needs to be treated with antibiotics, and most blocked ducts clear themselves without any treatment before the baby's first birthday. If your baby continues to have problems, talk to your doctor. I would normally refer a child with persistent blocked ducts to an ophthalmic surgeon to assess whether or not he or she needs an operation to open them.

WHAT YOU CAN DO

Take your baby to the doctor to confirm that the problem is blocked tear ducts. In the meantime, bathe the eye regularly with cotton wool dipped in cooled, boiled water. Use a separate piece of cotton wool for each stroke, and always wipe from the nose outwards. Gentle massage with a clean finger below the lower lid can also help.

Occasionally, if the secretions become infected, your baby may need antibiotic drops or ointment – your doctor will be able to provide you with advice.

▼ *Sticky eye caused by the build-up of natural secretions in the eye due to a blocked tear duct.*

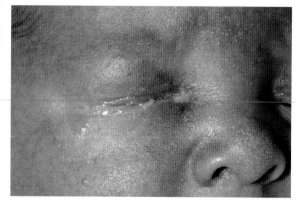

SQUINT

We expect our eyes to move together. When they don't move together, it can give the impression that a person is looking elsewhere when he or she is talking to you, or it's difficult to work out which eye is looking at you – this is called a squint and it happens because the muscles controlling the eye are not balanced.

WHO DOES IT AFFECT?

Squints are common, and affect around one in 50 children. The condition often runs in families, so if you are concerned talk to your doctor. If there is a family history of the condition, I would normally recommend that an optometrist do a full assessment on the child.

IS IT SERIOUS?

A child with a squint may stop using the affected eye, which can lead to visual loss if it's not treated. When babies are first born it is normal for their eyes to move independently of each other, but by the time they are three months old their eyes should be moving together. Sometimes, a baby just has a broad bridge to the nose, which can give the appearance of a squint that isn't actually there. If a squint is confirmed, your child may need to wear a patch over the good eye for a while, and he or she may need surgery to correct the muscles.

▼ *It may be necessary for an optometrist to carry out an assessment if your child has a squint.*

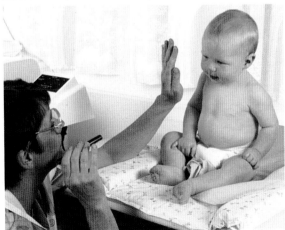

EAR INFECTIONS

A third of all children under three are taken to see their family doctor because of an infection in the middle ear (otitis media). Children born to mothers who smoked during pregnancy, who are bottle-fed, or who attend day nurseries are most at risk. Susceptibility also seems to run in families, so if you suffered as a child, the chances are your children may too.

WHY ARE THEY SO COMMON?

In babies and young children the tube that links the middle ear to the throat (the Eustachian tube) is relatively short, wide, and horizontal, so bugs can easily pass from the throat to the middle ear. As a child grows, this tube narrows and is pulled into a more vertical position, which is why middle-ear infections are much less common in older children and adults.

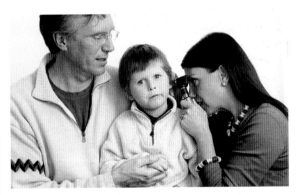

▲ *Ear infections are extremely common in young children.*

WHAT ARE THE SIGNS?

In the early stages, children with ear infections can often be grisly, and may have a fever. They may not be able to hear as well as usual, and they often tug at the ear or rub it. It is often more painful at night when the child is lying down.

Occasionally, the eardrum actually bursts and you will see a mucky or bloody discharge coming out of the ear. By the time this happens, you may be distraught at the sight of it, but your child is likely to be much more cheerful because the build-up of pressure is released.

ARE ANTIBIOTICS ESSENTIAL?

This is debatable. In fact, without antibiotics, around two-thirds of children will be feeling better after just 24 hours, and four out of five will be on the mend by day three. Serious complications such as meningitis are very rare in the Western world so it's not always necessary to use antibiotics early. I tend to reserve them for the children who are still suffering after several days, or who have a discharge. In the meantime, treat the pain and the fever – give your child plenty of fluids and the recommended doses of liquid paracetamol or ibuprofen.

HEARING LOSS

It's common for your child's hearing to be reduced for up to six weeks after an ear infection. Some children, however, develop an ongoing build-up of mucus in the middle ear called glue ear. This can lead to hearing problems for several months or years if not treated. To ensure normal language development, children with glue ear are often offered a hearing aid in the short term. Long-term treatment can involve an operation to insert small valves called grommets into the eardrum. If you are concerned about your child's hearing more than six weeks after an ear infection, talk to your doctor.

STAMMERING

Around one in 20 children under the age of five goes through a period when they stammer or stutter. Most of these children will grow out of it, developing normal speech.

WHAT YOU CAN DO

One in a hundred of these children is still stammering after the age of five. If left untreated, the stammering can persist into adulthood. Current thinking is that it is better to intervene early rather than late, as speech therapy can really help. So if you are concerned, talk to your doctor or health visitor about getting help.

HEARING LOSS

Babies will normally react to noise as soon as they are born, and hearing is extremely important for the development of speech and language skills in all children. Although rare, some babies are born with impaired hearing in one or both ears, and early detection is essential. In older children, it s more likely to be due to recurrent infections

TYPES OF HEARING LOSS

There are two main types of hearing loss:
• Conductive hearing loss – this type of hearing loss tends to affect low frequencies and is not usually severe. Common causes in children include wax in the ear canal, and infection or mucus build-up in the middle ear.
• Sensorineural hearing loss – this type of hearing loss is most frequently due to deterioration of the function of the inner ear as we age, but it can affect younger people too, particularly those exposed to excessive noise.

SHOULD I WORRY ABOUT MY CHILDREN USING PERSONAL MUSIC SYSTEMS?

More and more children seem to walk around with earphones in for several hours at a time and health professionals are concerned about possible long-term hearing damage. I have a simple rule with my children – if I can hear the bass, then it is too loud!

TREATMENT FOR HEARING LOSS

If you suspect your child may have hearing difficulty, you should take him or her to see your doctor, who will probably examine inside your child's ears. If an obvious cause can be found, such as wax or infection, this will be treated. Otherwise, your doctor will probably refer your child for special hearing tests to determine the extent and type of hearing loss. Depending on the results of these tests, a hearing aid may be recommended.

FIND OUT MORE
www.stammering.org

FIND OUT MORE
www.ndcs.org

HEAD LICE

These are small insects that can live on the scalp, laying eggs called nits. Infestations of head lice are very common, and they are spread by head-to-head contact, which is why they spread through nurseries and school so fast (and why children are sent home because of them).

AVOIDING HEAD LICE

One in five children has head lice at any one time, so catching them is relatively easy and getting rid of them can be surprisingly difficult.

The main problem is that head lice are becoming resistant to the chemicals used in insecticide lotions, so that even if the treatments are used properly and left on for 12 hours, some of the lice survive. There is also concern surrounding repeatedly using powerful lotions on children, especially as they are quite unpleasant to use and can be expensive. If you do want to use insecticide, there are different types available and it is important to alternate them. Talk to your pharmacist for advice, and it is worth bearing in mind that some are not recommended for use on children with asthma.

CHECK THE WHOLE FAMILY

As head lice are spread by direct contact, you won't necessarily need to treat everyone in the family but make sure you check everyone thoroughly, ideally

▼ *Working through the hair with fine-toothed nit comb remains an effective way to get rid of nits.*

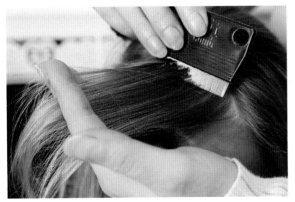

DR DAWN'S HEALTH CHECK
What you can do about head lice

There are number of ways to rid your child of lice without using chemicals, but given that a female louse lives for 30 days, laying about three eggs (nits) a day, and that each one will hatch in a week, this can take time. Perseverance is the name of the game.

• Wet combing – this is laborious but, in my opinion, the most effective treatment. Wash your child's hair, apply lots of conditioner to it, then work through the hair with a good old-fashioned fine-toothed nit comb. Pay particular attention to the nape of the neck and around the ears, where the lice congregate. You need to repeat this every day until you are sure the scalp is completely clear of lice and the nits.

• Natural insecticide – tea tree oil contains chemicals called monoterpenoids, which have an insecticide action, and some people find using the oil directly on the scalp is quite effective. Alternatively, make up your own solution. I was given a recipe by a friend of mine and it's worked on my kids: put 20 drops of tea tree oil and 20 drops of eucalyptus oil into 50ml (2fl oz) of a base oil (such as olive or sunflower). Massage the oil mixture liberally into the scalp and hair and leave on for at least an hour. Comb through with a nit comb and shampoo thoroughly; be prepared for this to take at least half an hour. Repeat the process every couple of days for at least a fortnight.

using the wet-combing method described in the box above. There is nothing more frustrating than spending hours ensuring one child is clear only to find that the next one is affected. Make sure affected children use separate towels, and wash all towels and bedding on a hot wash to kill any lice that have jumped ship.

FIND OUT MORE
www.headlice.org

TEETHING

There are no hard and fast rules as to when to expect your child's first teeth. Some children are born with teeth but most produce their first teeth (usually the middle ones on the lower gum) at around six months.

WHAT YOU SHOULD DO

Some babies seem to sail through teething with no symptoms at all, while others are grisly for a week or two before each tooth erupts, and may dribble excessively. You can buy teething gels that you rub on to the affected gum; alternatively, give him or her a cold teething ring to chew. Giving your baby the recommended dose of liquid paracetamol can also help.

DOES TEETHING CAUSE A FEVER?

No. Teething may make the child look red in the face and can coincide with an infection but will not cause a fever.

DOES TEETHING CAUSE NAPPY RASH?

Yes, or at least it can make a baby more prone to nappy rash. The theory is that some of the excess dribble is inevitably swallowed, which can lead to diarrhoea. Unless the nappy is changed immediately, sitting in a soiled nappy can cause a baby's bottom to become sore and so he or she is more likely to develop nappy rash.

▾ *Giving your baby a teething ring to chew on may help to alleviate some of the symptoms of teething.*

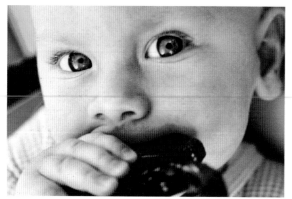

IMPETIGO

Nothing will get your child sent home from nursery or school faster than a bout of impetigo. It's a common infection that's caused by bacteria that live on your skin called *staphylococci*. Although it's not usually serious, impetigo does require treatment with antibiotics, either in the form of a cream or by mouth.

WHY DO SCHOOLS WORRY IF IT'S NOT SERIOUS?

Impetigo is highly contagious and it's spread by direct contact. Since toddlers and young children spend half their day hugging each other, if you allow a child with impetigo to stay at school the entire class could get it.

WHAT YOU SHOULD DO

If you suspect impetigo, take your child to your doctor sooner rather than later. If treated early, antibiotic cream is usually enough, but if it's left untreated the infected patch can become quite large and your child will almost certainly need oral antibiotics. Keep the spots as clean and dry as possible, don't let your child pick them, and make sure he or she has a separate flannel and towel. Wash the towel or facecloth thoroughly after use. Most cases of impetigo will clear within a week with the right treatment. Don't send your child back to school or nursery until all the spots have crusted over.

▾ *Impetigo causes blistering of the skin, most commonly around the mouth and nose.*

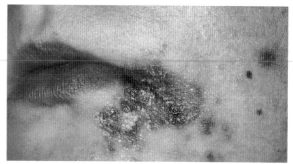

RASHES

Most children will develop rashes at some time and distinguishing between them or, worse, having to describe them, can be difficult if you don't happen to have a medical degree.

VIRAL RASH

Viral infections can cause a pink spotty rash that covers most of the body and can develop suddenly – I often see children who have gone to bed rash-free and woken up covered in spots. This type of rash tends to last a couple of days and then disappears. It is not usually serious and, in fact, often heralds the end of the other symptoms of the infection.

Managing the symptoms of the viral illness in the usual way with paracetamol and fluids is all that is usually needed. Viral rashes tend not to be itchy so shouldn't need any other treatment.

URTICARIA

This is the medical term for a raised, itchy, blotchy rash that makes your child look as if he or she has been stung by nettles. It is generally caused by allergy, usually to something your child has touched or eaten.

Antihistamine creams or syrup (depending on the extent of the rash) will help relieve the itching, but if

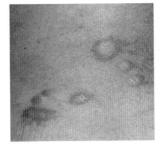

◀ *The rash of urticaria is typically raised, blotchy, and itchy.*

the rash is widespread and is getting worse, consult your doctor – in very severe cases urticaria may need treating with steroids.

ECZEMA AND PSORIASIS

It can be difficult to tell eczema and psoriasis apart (even for doctors), but as a general rule eczema tends to affect the inside (flexor) surfaces of the elbows and knees, while psoriasis is more likely to be on the outside (extensor) surfaces of these joints. See p.35 for advice on dealing with eczema, and p.36 for advice on dealing with psoriasis.

NAPPY RASH

The distribution of this rash, limited to the nappy area, makes it an easy diagnosis, but if left untreated it can become red and "angry". In the early stages, regular nappy changes, barrier creams, and time out of a nappy whenever practical should be all that is needed, but sometimes a secondary fungal infection will require special creams. If nappy rash isn't clearing up with simple measures, consult your health visitor or doctor.

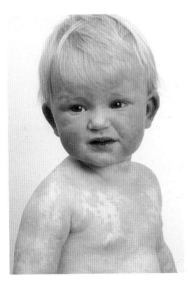

◀ *A viral infection may cause a pink rash that covers most of the body.*

> **! SEEK MEDICAL ADVICE NOW**
> **Meningitis**
> There are lots of different types of meningitis but the one that terrifies parents is meningococcal meningitis. Children with this condition are seriously ill and need urgent medical attention. The rash develops quickly all over the body and is deep red. It may start as spots but can rapidly develop into patches. Rolling a glass over the rash will not cause it to blanch – see next page.

MENINGITIS

A thin protective membrane called the meninges covers the brain and spinal cord. Meningitis simply means inflammation of this layer. Meningitis may be caused by a bacterial, viral, or fungal infection. The viral form is more common, but it is the bacterial form that is more severe, and can be life-threatening.

IS IT SERIOUS?

Yes – meningitis requires immediate medical attention and admission to hospital. Bacterial meningitis can cause seizures, drowsiness, and can lead to a coma unless treated promptly.

DO VACCINATIONS PROTECT AGAINST MENINGITIS?

Not against every type. All children in the UK are routinely offered immunization against pneumococcus and meningococcus type C. Most cases of meningitis in this country are caused by meningococcus types C and B, and work is being done to develop a type B vaccine.

IS IT INFECTIOUS?

Sometimes children will need antibiotics if they have been in contact with a child later diagnosed with meningitis. Meningitis is a notifiable disease; this means that the doctors who diagnose a case are obliged by law to inform the Public Health Department. The health authority will then contact anyone who is at risk of infection to make arrangements for them to have antibiotics as a precaution.

▼ *The red rash of meningococcal meningitis does not fade when pressed and viewed through a glass.*

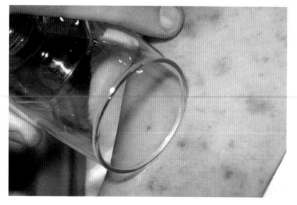

! SEEK MEDICAL ADVICE NOW

The symptoms of meningitis don't develop in any particular order, and may not all be present. Meningitis is a medical emergency, and if in doubt you should seek help immediately. If you can't contact your doctor, call an ambulance.

In a baby

It can be difficult to diagnose in very young babies. Trust your instincts – if you are concerned about your baby, get him or her to a doctor. Warning signs include:

- Floppy or fretful and possibly with a high-pitched cry.
- Loss of interest in food.
- Pale or blotchy skin.
- High fever but with cold hands and feet.
- Soft spot on top of the head (fontanelle) may be tense or bulging.
- Purple or red rash that does not fade if pressed.

In an older child

Symptoms in older children are easier to recognize and include:

- Flu-like illness with a high fever.
- Mottled or very pale skin.
- Cold hands and feet.

As the illness develops:

- Headache.
- Dislike of bright lights (photophobia).
- Neck stiffness.
- Vomiting.
- Drowsiness.
- Rash – the rash of meningococcal septicaemia doesn't fade under pressure. The glass test (see picture, left) is a good sign – roll the side of a glass over the rash. Most rashes disappear under the pressure, the rash of meningitis does not.

FIND OUT MORE

www.meningitis.uk
www.immunisation.nhs.uk

INFANTILE COLIC

If I had been paid extra for every mother I have ever seen in the surgery exhausted by a colicky baby, I would be sitting in the Caribbean right now. Colic is very common; as many as four in ten newborns suffer from it. Babies start to cry at the same time every day, usually in the evening, and it often starts when a baby is about three weeks old.

WHAT CAUSES IT?

No one knows what causes it, but the good news is that babies grow out of it by around 16 weeks. However, up to four months of interrupted evenings and sleepless nights can feel like a lifetime for the parents.

WHAT EXACTLY IS IT?

So what is colic? We don't really know. The term comes from the Greek word for colon, "*kolikos*", suggesting that it is due to a colon problem. Traditionally, doctors assumed that trapped gas was to blame but there is little evidence to support this. Some experts believe that the excess gas associated with colic is a symptom rather than a cause, arguing that crying babies swallow more air.

DR DAWN'S HEALTH CHECK
Tips for a colicky baby

If you have a colicky baby, you will no doubt be offered many solutions but here are a few tips worth trying:

• Studies have shown breast-fed babies are less likely to have colic, but watch your intake of coffee, alcohol, beans, onions, and spices. If you are bottle-feeding, try changing to a whey-hydrolysate formula.

• Playing soothing music, gently rocking your baby, and endless car rides in the dead of night worked for me, although there isn't any scientific evidence to support this.

• Anticolic preparations containing simethicone emulsion aren't scientifically proven to work but won't do any harm and do seem to help some babies.

• Laying your baby face down across your lap and rubbing his or her back can help.

DIARRHOEA AND VOMITING

Attacks of diarrhoea are common in children, especially those under the age of five. Most cases of diarrhoea and vomiting in children settle within 24 hours without specific treatment. However, it is essential that babies and young children have plenty of fluids, otherwise they can become dehydrated.

WHAT YOU CAN DO

The main concern when treating children is to make sure they are well hydrated. Give your child plenty of water to drink – over-the-counter rehydration preparations contain the ideal balance of salts and minerals and can be useful, but always check with your pharmacist that they are suitable for use in young children.

Young children who have had a stomach upset may develop a temporary intolerance to lactose, so giving your child milk diluted with boiled water (50:50) for a few days may help. If your child is hungry then it is fine to give them food as long as it doesn't make the symptoms any worse. As a general rule, keep it bland for the first few days.

SEEK MEDICAL ADVICE NOW
If your child:

• Has blood in the vomit or diarrhoea.

• Is becoming floppy and lifeless.

• Has a high fever.

• Has dry nappies – a sign that he or she is becoming dehydrated.

• Symptoms that persist for more than 24 hours, or become worse.

• Has projectile vomiting and is under six weeks old. Adults tend to wretch and vomit with force. In babies, the muscular opening (sphincter) between the bottom of the gullet and the stomach is less well developed, so when they vomit they are often producing overflow from the stomach. However, violent vomiting in a very young baby could indicate that there is a narrowing at the stomach exit, which must be checked by a doctor.

CONSTIPATION

This is surprisingly common in children – hardly a week goes by without a child with constipation being brought to see me. Children will all differ in their bowel habits, but around one in ten children will get constipated at some time.

WHEN IS IT A PROBLEM?

When your baby is still in nappies you are only too aware of how often he or she opens his or her bowels, but as soon as the child is potty trained it's one delight that most of us don't give too much thought to, and most of the time it doesn't matter.

The problem begins when a child becomes "bunged up". Hard faeces can be more difficult, and sometimes even painful, to pass. A child's natural reaction to the discomfort is to avoid opening his or her bowels, so the stool just gets even larger and harder. Before you know it, your child is struggling with tummy-ache and a sore bottom. In extreme cases, children may even suffer from leaking from a more liquid stool above the hard one. Parents often mistake this for diarrhoea.

WHAT YOU CAN DO

Like most things, prevention is better than cure – ensure that your child gets plenty of exercise, eats a high-fibre diet, and drinks plenty of fluids, then you should avoid the problem.

But if despite this your child is still having difficulty, talk to your pharmacist. There are plenty of gentle laxatives available for children, some with a pleasant syrupy taste, which always makes life easier. Don't be surprised if your child needs laxatives for several months as it can take a long time to re-establish a regular bowel routine, but don't worry, your child's system won't become dependent on them.

THREADWORMS

The threadworm is the most common worm that can live in the human body. Infection with threadworms are very common in children – almost half of all ten-year-olds will have had at least one infestation.

WHAT ARE THE SYMPTOMS?

Although the adult worms only live for six weeks, the female worms lay their eggs (ova) on the skin around the bottom at night, causing itching. Children in particular scratch the area in their sleep, which leads to the ova being transmitted on the fingers to the mouth, often via food eaten with unwashed hands.

WHAT YOU CAN DO

Washing hands and scrubbing nails before each meal and after every visit to the toilet will help prevent transmission. It is also a good idea to give your child a bath or shower first thing in the morning, asking him or her to take extra care to wash around the bottom to remove any eggs laid the night before.

Give your child a threadworm treatment available from the chemist. Choose a preparation containing piperazine. It is taken as a one-off dose and will eradicate the worms, but as reinfestation is so common it is worth repeating the dose a fortnight later. Wash all bedding and towels on a hot wash after the treatment.

▼ Teaching children good hand hygiene helps prevent the spread of threadworms.

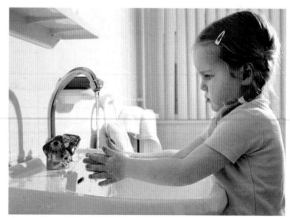

FADDY EATING

Some children are always more adventurous with food than others. Researchers have found that children seem to have a window in their development between the ages of about six and nine months when they are more likely to accept new foods. Introducing a range of flavours and textures at this stage may help to prevent faddy eating in later life.

WHAT YOU CAN DO

If, like I did, you spend hours at the liquidizer trying to convert all the elements of your balanced meal into the perfect purée, then think again. It's often better to keep the components of the meal separate, and to leave them with some texture. That way your child can log each texture and taste, which could go a long way to broadening his or her palate for the future.

If the faddy eating persists, try not to make meal times a battleground, as this will only make things worse. Most children will grow out of it in their own time.

▾ Faddy eating habits are quite common in young children but most eventually grow out of them.

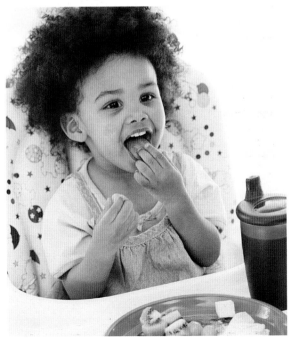

APPENDICITIS

This is inflammation of a small finger-shaped tube that branches off the large intestine. Appendicitis is so common that around one in six children will have their appendix removed before adulthood. However, it can be surprisingly difficult to make the diagnosis; nearly half of the children operated on are found not to have appendicitis at all.

IS IT SERIOUS?

If an inflamed appendix is left alone it may perforate, causing peritonitis (inflammation of the abdominal wall), which can be fatal. Although no one wants unnecessary surgery, when it comes to appendicitis it is often better to be safe than sorry.

HOW CAN YOU TELL IF IT'S APPENDICITIS

Appendicitis usually starts as a colicky pain around the navel and only moves to the site you associate with appendicitis – the bottom right corner of the abdomen – after about six hours. Children with appendicitis find that moving makes the pain worse and they often lie still with their knees bent up in a fetal position. They are invariably off their food and some children will be sick. A child with appendicitis nearly always has a fever and looks flushed; and if you touch his or her abdomen around the area of the appendix, it will be very tender.

SEEK MEDICAL ADVICE

If your child has abdominal pain and you think it could be appendicitis, get him or her to a doctor. Importantly, don't give your child anything to eat or drink just in case he or she needs surgery. The good news is that the majority of appendectomies are done using keyhole surgery, so children recover very quickly – most will be out of hospital and on the road to recovery within a couple of days.

GROWING PAINS

People used to talk about growing pains a lot a generation or so ago, but it's a diagnosis you rarely hear today. So do growing pains exist? I believe they do and they are more common than you might think – as many as one in four children suffers from them, either between the ages of three and five or between eight and 12.

WHAT ARE THE SIGNS?

Classically, children complain of aching in their thighs or calves, usually at night, and they last for around half an hour. The pains tend to occur several times a week for a few weeks and then disappear for a while, and are often worse after very active days. Doctors don't fully understand what causes the pains, but you only have to watch the average ten-year-old child race around all day to understand why their muscles might just complain at the end of the day. As long as your child doesn't experience the pain during the day and has no swelling or bruising, then there is unlikely to be a more serious underlying cause.

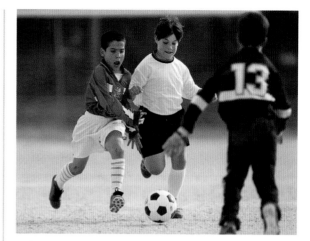

▲ Growing pains are common in children, especially after vigorous physical activity.

WHAT YOU CAN DO

The treatment is simple – give the recommended dose of liquid paracetamol, reassurance, gentle massage on the affected area, and lots of cuddles.

WILL THE PAINS STOP?

The good news is that most children literally grow out of these pains within a couple of years. There is some evidence to indicate that children who are very restless with the pain are at a greater risk of developing restless leg syndrome in adulthood (see p.115).

> **? DID YOU KNOW**
> ### Childhood limping
> The gait of a child is different from that of an adult during their first three years. Their balance is not yet fully developed so to compensate they take a lot more steps and walk at a slower speed. In an attempt to lower their centre of gravity and improve balance, they also flex their hips, knees, and ankles more than adults.
>
> When your child walks, 60 per cent of the time will involve having their feet on the ground and transmitting body weight, so anything causing pain from the hip down can result in a limp. All children will limp occasionally and usually the cause is obvious, but a child who limps for no apparent reason must be seen by a doctor. If you are not sure why your child is suddenly limping, take their temperature and if it is raised get them to a doctor straight away. It could be a sign of an infection in the joint (septic arthritis) – this is an emergency that will need aggressive treatment with antibiotics in hospital to prevent long-term problems.

> **! SEEK MEDICAL ADVICE NOW**
> **If your child develops any of the following:**
> • Pain in only one leg or in a joint.
> • Pain lasting hours.
> • Limping for no obvious reason.
> • Redness or swelling.
> • Fever or rash.

NAIL BITING

This is rarely serious enough to warrant a trip to the doctor in its own right (although I do occasionally see children with secondary infections caused by nail biting or others who have damaged the nail bed so badly they have lost the nail). But parents often ask me how they should deal with it.

IS IT COMMON?

Nail biting is very common. Occasionally, it's a sign that a child has anxiety problems, for most it's just a bad habit.

Children usually start nail biting from about three years old. By the time they reach their teens, about half of them bite their nails. Most kick the habit in their twenties if not before – only one in ten people over 35 are nail biters.

WHAT YOU CAN DO

Simple remedies, such as painting the nails with a bitter-tasting substance like mustard, work for some, but for older children behavioural therapies, aimed at relaxation and self-control, may be more effective. If done properly, these help as many as four in every ten stop completely, and another four will significantly reduce their habit.

As a parent, look for some sort of positive reward or bribe – for girls having prettier hands may be enough, but for boys you will probably have to be a bit more inventive.

▾ Nail biting is very common in children and is something that most will grow out of by the time they reach their twenties.

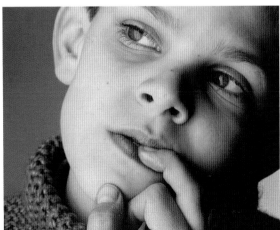

POTTY TRAINING

Children need to be able to understand and follow simple instructions before they can be potty trained. Boys tend to learn control later than girls, but as a rough guide most children are dry during the day by the time they are three years old and at night by the age of four – although five per cent of ten-year-olds still wet the bed, so there is a huge variation.

HOW DO YOU KNOW A CHILD IS READY?

The key to successful potty training is to wait until your child is ready. Indications that a child is ready to start training include:

- Showing an interest in others using the toilet and wanting to copy them.
- Playing with the potty.
- Talking about "poo".
- Being dry between nappy changes.

Some children seem to learn what to do in only a few days, while others take months and have several relapses on the way.

WHAT YOU CAN DO

Get a potty some time before the child is ready, and tell him or her what it's for. When your child starts showing signs that he or she is ready, take their daytime nappy off when you are at home. Congratulate your child if he or she manages to use the potty. If it doesn't work initially, put the nappy back on and try again in a week or so.

Waiting until your child is ready is essential for successful potty training. ▸

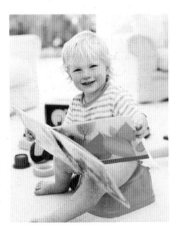

BEDWETTING

This is surprisingly common – 15 per cent of five-year-olds and five per cent of ten-year-olds still wet their beds at night. Most will grow out of it even if they are still having accidents in their teens – only one in 100 adults has problems, but that's not much consolation if it's your washing machine that is about to give up the ghost, or your ten-year-old child who is too embarrassed to go to a sleepover.

YOUR DOCTOR MAY BE ABLE TO HELP

If my tips don't work, then talk to your doctor. He or she will make sure that there is no medical reason for the bedwetting and may suggest trying an enuresis alarm. The child has a sensor in the bed, or attached to nightwear, which is linked to an alarm. The alarm sounds at the first sign of wetness, waking the child, who can then get up and go to the loo. Children are 13 times more likely to succeed with an alarm than without one.

There are also several drug treatments available, some of which can be used on a one-off basis, so don't let bedwetting stop your child staying over with friends.

Just one word of warning, though – if a child has been dry at night for a long while and suddenly starts wetting the bed, it can be a sign of emotional distress.

DR DAWN'S HEALTH CHECK
Encouraging dry nights

There are a few simple measures you can take that may help:

• Don't give your child fluids late at night but encourage daytime drinks. Five or six extra cups of water during the day can help to increase the bladder capacity.

• Cut out caffeine as it's a diuretic – remember it's in cola drinks not just tea and coffee.

• Avoid blackcurrant drinks as they can irritate the bladder in susceptible children.

• Treat constipation as it can increase pressure on the bladder.

• Try a star chart – they are surprisingly successful.

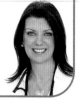

CHILDHOOD DEPRESSION

In the last ten years I have seen a rise in the number of children coming through my surgery door with depression. It is rare in young children, but as many as one in 20 adolescents has significant symptoms of depression and many more will show some features of the illness.

WHAT ARE THE SIGNS?

Often the classic signs of being withdrawn, angry, tearful, and uncommunicative, as any parent of a teen will tell you, are all part of normal teenage behaviour. But there are telltale signs to look out for: the child who suddenly does less well at school, who never concentrates on anything, or who loses interest in hobbies and social life would raise alarm bells for me.

TREATMENT

It is vital that you keep trying to communicate and if possible get him or her to your doctor. Many antidepressants are not recommended for children, but the talking therapies like cognitive behavioural therapy (see p.180) can work wonders.

▾ Childhood depression has become increasingly common.

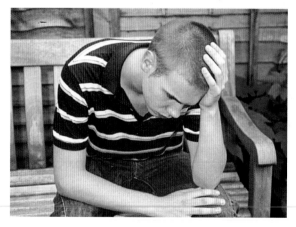

FIND OUT MORE
www.youngminds.co.uk

ADHD

Attention deficit hyperactivity disorder (ADHD) is one of the most common disorders of childhood; it affects as many as one in 20 children – that's half a million children in the UK alone. It is four times more common in boys, but although boys with ADHD tend to be more hyperactive and disruptive, girls often show symptoms such as poor attention span.

THERE IS A GENETIC LINK

The genetic link is so strong that if a family has one child with ADHD, there is a 30 to 40 per cent chance that another child will have the condition. If an ADHD child has an identical twin, there is a 90 per cent chance that the other twin will have it too.

DOES IT JUST AFFECT CHILDREN?

Doctors used to think ADHD was a only disorder of childhood, and that it was something children grew out of. It is now known that two-thirds of sufferers will continue to have problems into adulthood. It is often less obvious in adults because they learn how to cope with their symptoms.

HOW IS ADHD DIAGNOSED?

Most children show occasional ADHD traits, but the true ADHD child is consistently hyperactive or inattentive in all social settings, whether at home, with friends, or at school. A specialist should always make the diagnosis. It's important to identify the problem as early as possible because the sooner treatment is started, the better the outcome.

TREATMENT

Most experts agree that the most effective treatment involves a combination of psychological therapy, family therapy, educational modifications and, for the most severe cases, medication that alters the levels of chemicals in the brain. Some parents find an improvement when foods such as chocolate, cola, and artificial colourings are excluded from a child's diet. Drug treatment is reserved for the most severe cases.

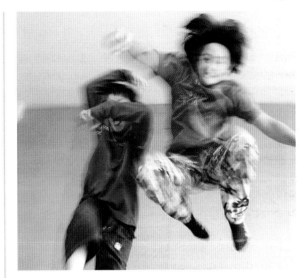

▲ *Constant hyperactivity in all social settings could indicate ADHD.*

Paradoxically, the drugs we use are designed to be psychological stimulants, and when used in adults they make people more alert and awake. In ADHD children, they have the opposite effect, producing significant improvement in attention and concentration. Parents often tell me that they notice a difference within just half an hour of giving the medicine.

WHAT IF MY DOCTOR WON'T PRESCRIBE MEDICATION?

Doctors are not allowed to start medication for ADHD until the condition has been diagnosed by a specialist after a full assessment. However, your doctor may be happy to issue repeat prescriptions after its initiation.

ARE THERE ANY SIDE EFFECTS?

Parents are often worried about giving stimulant drugs to developing brains, but most children have very few side effects. It can cause sleep problems and a reduced appetite which has raised concerns over growth, but it is not generally affected.

FIND OUT MORE
www.addiss.co.uk

LEARNING DIFFICULTIES

About two in every 100 children in the UK have learning difficulties, and there is a wide variation in what we mean by this. Strictly speaking, the term "learning disability" refers to below-average IQ, but it is often used to include those with specific disorders, often related to numeracy, reading and writing.

DIAGNOSING LEARNING DIFFICULTIES

A small minority of parents know that their child will have developmental problems when they are first born. For the majority, the realization that their son or daughter may have difficulties is a gradual process which takes months, or sometimes years, to come to light.

If you do have concerns over your child's development, it is better to ask for help sooner rather than later. If there are problems, then the sooner these are addressed, the sooner you will get the appropriate support network in place, and the greater your child's chance will be of reaching his or her full potential.

As a rough guide, children with an IQ of 50–70 are considered to have mild difficulties, while an IQ of below 20 is associated with profound disability.

WHAT HAPPENS NEXT?

If your child is diagnosed with learning difficulties, there are two questions that you will probably want to ask – why has this happened, and what does the future hold?

Your child may have a chromosome abnormality, or there may have been an event around the birth resulting in them not receiving enough oxygen. However, quite often there may not be a reason, and dwelling on it can be unhelpful. Health professionals are often reluctant to predict if your child will go to mainstream school or hold down a job and that's because IQ isn't the whole picture – personality and support play a huge role in how your child will develop.

FIND OUT MORE
www.mencap.org.uk

CHILDHOOD IMMUNIZATIONS

The childhood immunization programme is aimed at protecting as many children as possible from serious infectious diseases. By giving a vaccination, the child develops antibodies to that disease. If they then come into contact with the infection in later life their immune system can fight it off. Most vaccinations are given to young babies in order to give protection as early as possible.

ARE THEY SAFE?

All children in the UK who are registered with a National Health doctor are routinely offered immunizations at two, three, four, 12, and 13 months (see opposite). Of course, whether or not you take up the offer is entirely down to personal choice. I meet a lot of parents who are worried about possible side effects of vaccinations, and of course nothing is risk-free in life, but the bottom line for me is that modern vaccinations are safer than ever, but the diseases they protect against are not.

▼ *The childhood immunization schedule in the UK starts at the age of two months and continues into the teens.*

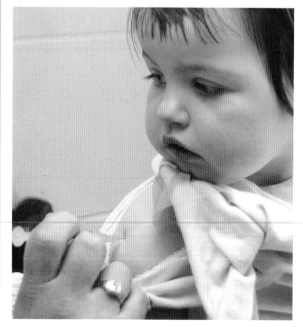

WHY IS IMMUNIZATION ONLY STARTED WHEN A BABY IS TWO MONTHS OLD?

If a vaccination is given to someone who has antibodies to the disease already, their immune system will not take it up.

All babies receive antibodies from their mothers during pregnancy via the placenta. These antibodies remain in the baby's immune system for up to two months, after which time they are lost. Therefore, two months is the earliest age you can be sure that the vaccines will work effectively.

MY BABY WAS PREMATURE, SHOULD I DELAY THE FIRST VACCINES?

No, definitely not. Premature babies are at higher risk of infection so they must be immunized quickly.

SHOULD I POSTPONE THE IMMUNIZATION IF MY BABY HAS A COLD?

No. A cough or cold is not a reason to delay vaccination. If, however, your child has a temperature, then giving the injection could make this worse and it is sensible to delay until the fever subsides. If in doubt, take your child along

THE UK IMMUNIZATION SCHEDULE

All children in the UK are routinely offered the following vaccinations. As long as you are registered with a National Health doctor, you don't have to remember to make the appointments, the surgery or baby clinic will contact you.

Age	Immunization	Date your child is immunized
Two months old	Diphtheria, tetanus, whooping cough, haemophilus influenzae (one injection) and polio (drop) Pneumococcal infection (one injection)	
Three months old	Diphtheria, tetanus, whooping cough, haemophilus influenzae (one injection) and polio (drop) Meningitis C (one injection)	
Four months old	Diphtheria, tetanus, whooping cough, haemophilus influenzae (one injection) and polio (drop) Pneumococcal infection (one injection) Meningitis C (one injection)	
12 months old	Haemophilus influenzae and meningitis C (one injection)	
13 months old	Measles, mumps, rubella – MMR (one injection) Pneumococcal infection (one injection)	
Between three years four months and five years old	Diphtheria, tetanus, whooping cough (one injection) and polio (drop) Measles, mumps, and rubella – MMR (one injection)	
Between 13 and 18 years old	Diphtheria, tetanus (one injection) and polio (drop)	

to your clinic appointment and ask the doctor to check him or her over before giving the vaccine.

IS THERE DANGER OF OVERLOADING YOUNG CHILDREN WITH VACCINES?

This is probably the most commonly asked question in our baby clinic, and the answer is absolutely not. Babies are exposed to literally thousands of bacteria and viruses on a daily basis, all of which challenge their immune systems. In theory, a baby's immune system could cope with 10,000 vaccines at one time and your child is given a maximum of six in one go, so we are a long way off overloading them.

CAN MY BABY HAVE MEASLES, MUMPS, AND RUBELLA AS SEPARATE INJECTIONS?

Because of the recent discussion about the single measles, mumps, and rubella (MMR) vaccine, there has been a lot of interest in single vaccines. However, they are not licensed in the UK and there is no evidence that they are any safer. In fact, there is an argument that giving the injections separately could put children at increased risk of developing measles, mumps, or rubella in the gaps between them. I still believe that giving the MMR at 13 months and as a preschool booster is the safest way to protect your children from the diseases, and that's what I did with my children.

FIND OUT MORE
www.mmrthefacts.phs.uk
www.immunization.nhs.uk

CHICKENPOX

This disease is caused by infection with a herpes virus called varicella zoster. The rash is quite distinctive in that each spot has three stages: it starts as a pink spot, which rapidly becomes a blister, and then it crusts over. The difference between chickenpox spots and any other type of rash is that there will be spots at all stages of development present at the same time.

HOW LONG IS A CHILD INFECTIOUS?

Chickenpox spreads from person to person, either via droplets in the air or by direct contact with broken blisters, which are literally teeming with the virus. It can take anything from ten to 20 days after contracting the virus for the rash to develop. A child is infectious from about three days before the rash appears until the last blister has scabbed over.

IS CHICKENPOX MORE SERIOUS FOR ADULTS?

Yes. Chickenpox lasts about seven to ten days in children but can last a lot longer in adults, who are also more likely to suffer the more serious complications, such as chickenpox pneumonitis – a potentially fatal chest infection that causes you to cough up blood and which requires urgent medical attention.

WHAT YOU CAN DO

Chickenpox affects children in different ways – some sail through looking dreadful, but seemingly unbothered by the spots, while others are driven mad with itching. Give recommended doses of liquid paracetamol to help control any fever. Dab the spots with calamine lotion, and give antihistamine syrup if the spots are very itchy. Keep your child's fingernails cut short to minimize any damage to the skin from scratching. If your child is severely affected, or is known to have a weak immune system, consult your doctor.

SHOULD A CHILD WITH CHICKENPOX STAY AWAY FROM FRIENDS?

Not necessarily. However, your child should avoid contact with pregnant women as the chickenpox virus can harm

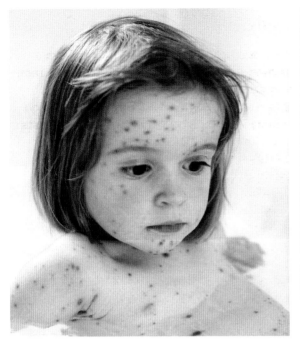

▲ *Chickenpox is infectious from about three days before the rash appears until the last blister has scabbed over.*

an unborn baby if the mother hasn't had chickenpox. Babies are also at risk of severe attacks of chickenpox if exposed to the virus. It is also important to stay away from anyone whose immune system is weakened, such as those undergoing chemotherapy, those who have AIDS, or those with leukaemia.

? **DID YOU KNOW**
Catching chickenpox from shingles

When you have chickenpox, your body never completely clears the virus – it travels back down the nerve endings and lies dormant near your spinal cord.

The virus can be activated again if your immune system is low, for example if you are very stressed, when it appears as shingles, a painful rash of tiny blisters that appear in bands across your back or abdomen. This rash contains the active virus and anyone not immune to the virus could develop chickenpox. However, the reverse is not the case – you can't catch shingles from someone with chickenpox.

GLANDULAR FEVER

Glandular fever, also referred to as the "kissing disease", is mainly spread through saliva. It can be caught by anyone, although it is most common among teenagers. The classic symptoms are fever, sore throat, painful swollen glands, and general fatigue. These symptoms usually follow a week or two after infection but the incubation period can be as long as seven weeks.

HOW DO YOU TREAT GLANDULAR FEVER?

Glandular fever is caused by a virus called Epstein-Barr virus and won't respond to treatment with antibiotics. Drinking plenty of fluids and taking paracetamol or aspirin is the best treatment. Rest is essential, and contact sports must be avoided because glandular fever causes an enlarged spleen.

CHRONIC FATIGUE SYNDROME

Around one in 20 people suffer from prolonged fatigue following glandular fever, which sometimes lasts for several months. Normally, individuals make complete recovery from the acute symptoms within a month, with a gradual return to normal energy levels.

▼ *Glandular fever causes fever, sore throat, painful swollen glands, and general fatigue.*

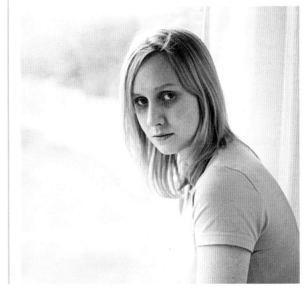

MEASLES

This is a serious and highly contagious viral disease spread by droplet infection. Immunization is offered to all children in the UK in the MMR vaccine.

WHAT ARE THE SYMPTOMS?

If a child is in contact with measles, it takes about 14 days for the symptoms of fever, sore throat, and cough to develop.

What distinguishes measles from a simple sore throat is the greyish spots that appear inside the mouth around the molar teeth, called Koplik's spots. Just after these spots form, the typical pink measles rash starts to develop. It usually begins as a fine rash around the ears' but over the course of a couple of days the spots enlarge and spread all over the body. Your child should hopefully recover after a week, but shouldn't return to school until the fever and rash are gone.

WHAT YOU CAN DO

Treatment will involve a lot of tender loving care, liquid paracetamol to help control the fever, and bed rest in a cool room. If you cannot control the fever, or your child develops a cough or severe earache, then see your doctor.

▼ *The pink rash of measles starts around the ears then spreads all over the body within a couple of days.*

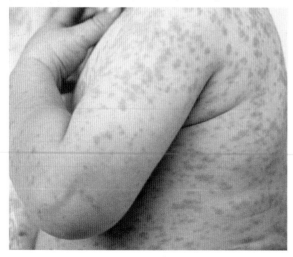

MUMPS

This is caused by a virus known as paramyxovirus, which is spread via droplets in the air. It can take three weeks from infection to the development of fever and swollen glands around the jaw that gives the classic "chipmunk" look.

WHAT YOU CAN DO

Children with mumps should stay in bed and rest until the fever and swelling have settled. Give the recommended dose of liquid paracetamol to control the fever.

HOW LIKELY ARE COMPLICATIONS?

The older the child is, the more likely he or she is to develop complications such as meningitis (see p.216) or orchitis (swelling and inflammation of the testicles). If a man has mumps, there is a 20–30 per cent chance that he will develop orchitis, which can lead to problems with fertility.

▼ *Mumps causes swollen glands around the jaw, here affecting mainly the right side of the face.*

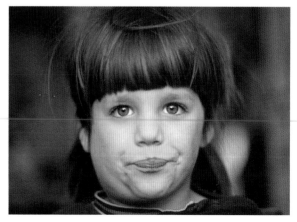

RUBELLA

Also know as German measles, this is another virus infection also spread by droplets in the air. There can be three weeks between contracting the virus and developing the classic symptoms of a mild flu-like illness followed by a pink rash, which typically spreads from behind the ears to all over the body within a few hours.

IS RUBELLA SERIOUS?

Your child may not be very unwell with rubella, but it can have a devastating effect on unborn babies. All UK children registered with a National Health doctor are offered a vaccine against rubella (as part of the MMR). You only have to see the result of one case of rubella caught during pregnancy, leaving a baby blind, deaf, and mentally handicapped, to understand the importance of the immunization programme.

WHAT YOU CAN DO

If your child contracts rubella, he or she won't need any specific treatment other than rest, plenty of fluids, and liquid paracetamol. While your child is infectious, it's essential to keep him or her away from pregnant women and anyone with a weakened immune system. A child is at his or her most infectious when the rash is at its peak. But they can pass the infection on any time from a week before the rash develops until a week after it has gone. If you have to take your child to your doctor, tell the surgery in advance that you suspect rubella.

▾ *Rubella causes a pink rash that spreads all over the body within a matter of hours.*

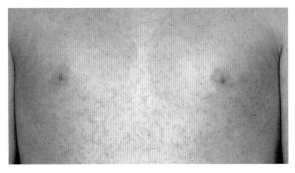

WHOOPING COUGH

Whooping cough, also known as pertussis, is caused by a bacterium. It usually begins as a mild cough but rapidly develops, clogging the airways with mucus and causing the severe coughing bouts that gave it its name. These coughing bouts can occur up to 50 times a day for as long as eight weeks.

WHAT YOU CAN DO

Most cases of whooping cough require no specific treatment, but if your child suffers from asthma your doctor will want to keep a close eye on him or her.

Whooping cough, because it is a bacterial infection, may be treated with antibiotics in the early stages to prevent it from spreading, particularly if the diagnosis is made early on. After five days of antibiotics, your child will no longer be infectious, but if left untreated he or she could pass on the infection for several weeks.

▾ *Whooping cough causes the airways to clog with mucus, and can cause severe coughing bouts.*

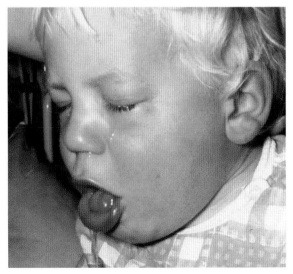

- Most accidents happen in the home, so you are much more likely to use first aid to treat someone you know rather than a stranger • It takes three to four minutes for a blocked airway to kill someone, so it is really important to know what to do while you wait for help to arrive – it may help to save a life • Around half of all people attending accident and emergency departments in the UK have minor injuries or illnesses, many of which could have been managed at home • First aid training courses are widely available – a short course of just three hours may give you the knowledge and confidence to deal with an emergency.

20

First aid

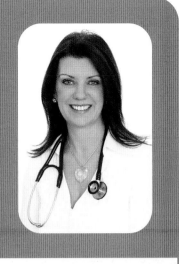

HOME FIRST AID KIT

Every home should have a first aid kit. You will never be able to equip yourself for all emergencies, but a few basics are essential for dealing with the things you are most likely to encounter. It is a good idea to keep a first aid kit in your car as well. Check any medicines regularly to make sure they are not out of date. As a guide, I would advise making sure that you always have the following in stock:

HOME EQUIPMENT

- Plasters in an assortment of sizes.
- Special blister plasters.
- Sterile dressings in an assortment of sizes.
- Triangular bandage and safety pins.
- Roller bandages – you'll need at least two; choose the compression bandages as they mould to the shape of the limb.
- Hypoallergenic tape for securing dressings.
- Non-alcoholic wound cleaning wipes.
- Sterile eye wash.

- Disposable gloves – to protect yourself from body fluids. Keep both latex and plastic gloves as some people are allergic to latex.
- Scissors – preferably round-ended so they will not cause any injuries.
- Tweezers.
- Digital thermometer.

HOME MEDICINES

- Paracetamol – in liquid form if you have children, and as tablets.
- Anti-inflammatory medication – for example, ibuprofen; in liquid form if you have children, and as tablets.
- Antihistamines – as cream and tablets, and in syrup form if you have children.
- Antiseptic cream.
- Indigestion remedy (for adults).

EXTRA EQUIPMENT FOR YOUR CAR

- Warning triangle.
- Survival blanket.
- Notebook and pen.
- Spare mobile phone, if you have one – don't forget to keep it charged.

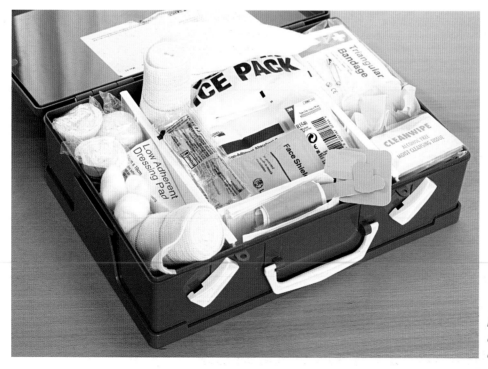

◀ *First aid kits can be bought ready made up or you can put together one yourself.*

BASIC PRINCIPLES

One situation that most people dread is witnessing someone collapse. Keeping your cool and knowing what to do next really could save a life. I think everyone should be trained in basic first aid, but I am well aware that learning in a classroom is very different from a real-life situation. Using "ABC" as a simple reminder of what to do next will help you to think clearly and act quickly,

A IS FOR AIRWAY

Ensuring a clear airway is an essential first step in resuscitation. Tilt the casualty's head back, which will cause the mouth to fall open. Remove any obvious obstructions from the mouth (such as broken teeth or dentures). Do not remove well-fitting dentures and do not sweep your finger around the casualty's mouth. Next lift the casualty's chin and check if the casualty is breathing.

B IS FOR BREATHING

To check if the casualty is breathing, look at the chest to see if it is rising and falling as you would expect; listen for sounds of breathing; and place your cheek close to the mouth to feel for breath.

C IS FOR CIRCULATION

If you are going to achieve a successful resuscitation you not only need to deliver oxygen to the lungs via a clear airway, you also need to get the heart pumping blood, so checking the circulation is vital. To do this, kneel by the casualty's head and look, listen, and feel for signs of circulation, such as breathing, coughing, or movement.

See pages 240–241 for information on how to administer cardiopulmonary resucitation (CPR).

> **FIND OUT MORE**
> www.redcross.gov.uk
> www.firstaid.org.uk
> www.sja.org.uk

TAKING A TEMPERATURE

Normal body temperature for most people is 37°C (98.6°F). However, normal for some people may be slightly above or below this, so it's worth knowing yours and your family's when well, and it's therefore important to know how to take a temperature properly.

TYPES OF THERMOMETER

Digital thermometers are probably the best for home use and are not expensive. Doctors tend to use infrared ear (aural) thermometers, which are accurate and quick and easy to use but can be very expensive. The traditional glass mercury thermometers are reliable but can be difficult to read and are no longer readily available because mercury is being phased out. I would also avoid the strips that stick on the forehead because they just aren't accurate enough.

USING A DIGITAL THERMOMETER

Sit yourself (or your child) down quietly. Switch on the thermometer, place it under the tongue, and wait until it beeps – it should take about a minute.

For a young child, it is safer and easier to measure the temperature by putting the thermometer in his or her armpit. Hold the child's arm while it is recording (it may take two to three minutes); then add 0.5°C (1°F) to the reading to obtain the child's body temperature.

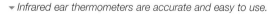

▼ *Infrared ear thermometers are accurate and easy to use.*

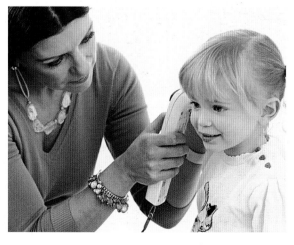

CHOKING

Food or small objects can get stuck in the back of the throat, blocking it, or cause spasm of the muscles around the throat. If the blockage is partial, the person may be able to clear it him- or herself. If the blockage is total, they will need help.

1 If the person can still speak, cough, and breathe, the obstruction is probably only partial, and simply encouraging him or her to cough may be all that is needed to clear the airway.

2 If the person is unable to speak or cough, you will need to help them. Bend them forwards and support him or her with one hand. Give five sharp blows on his or her back between the shoulder blades with the heel of your hand to try to dislodge the obstruction. Check the mouth after each back blow.

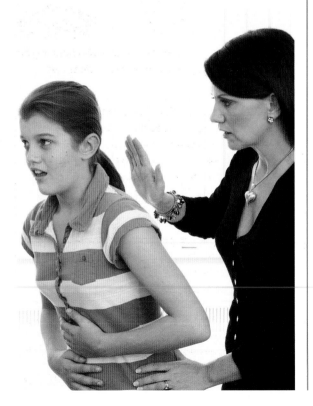

3 If this fails to clear the airway, stand behind the person and put your arms around the upper abdomen. Place one fist, thumb inwards, against the person's abdomen between the navel and the bottom of his or her chest. Cover the fist with your other hand, then pull sharply inwards and upwards – this is called an abdominal thrust. Repeat this five times. Check the mouth again.

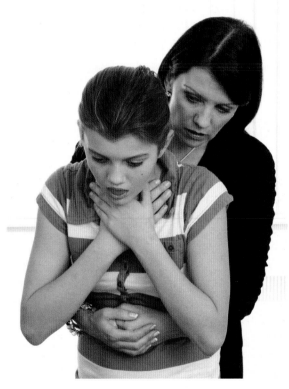

4 If you still have not cleared the airway, repeat steps 2 and 3 up to three times.

 EMERGENCY – DIAL 999

If after three cycles of back slaps and abdominal thrusts, you have not succeeded in clearing the airway, either ask someone to call an ambulance, or stop and do it yourself. Continue alternating back slaps and abdominal thrusts until the ambulance arrives. If the person loses consciousness, carry out the steps on p.240.

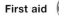

BLEEDING

Always wear disposable gloves when you are dealing with open wounds to protect yourself from infection. It's important to keep wounds clean to prevent an infection developing later.

MINOR CUTS AND GRAZES

Clean the injury. Holding the injury under cold running water is often enough. If you have no water to hand, use non-alcoholic wound cleaning wipes instead. Then dab the area dry with a clean, non-fluffy cloth and cover the wound with a sterile dressing or plaster to protect it (the dressing area must be larger than the wound).

MORE SERIOUS BLEEDING

• Control the bleeding by applying pressure to the wound, ideally over a sterile pad. Raise the affected part above the level of the casualty's heart to slow down the blood flow to the injury. Serious bleeding is likely to make the casualty feel faint, so help him or her to lie down but keep the injury raised.

• Put a bandage over the sterile pad to keep pressure on the injury. This needs to be firm enough to maintain the direct pressure on the bleeding but not so tight that it cuts off the circulation to the area beyond it.

• If blood starts to show through the first bandage, put another pad and bandage on top. If it comes through the second bandage, the direct pressure is probably not in the right place; in this case, remove all the bandages and start again.

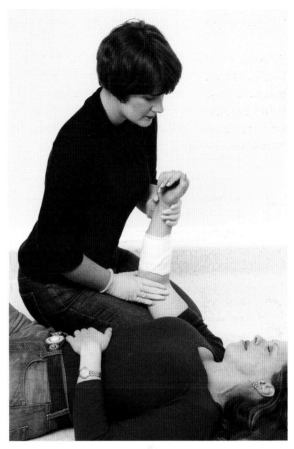

▲ More serious bleeding can often be controlled by raising the wounded area and applying pressure over a sterile pad.

> **! EMERGENCY – DIAL 999**
>
> Severe bleeding is an emergency. You may be able to take the casualty to the nearest accident and emergency department yourself, although you should not move the casualty but should call an ambulance if:
> • You have no one to help you support the casualty while you drive.
> • There is an object embedded in the wound.
> • The casualty is impaled on an object.

> **DR DAWN'S HEALTH CHECK**
> **Dealing with an embedded object**
>
> If an object is embedded in a wound, your aims are to control bleeding without pressing on the object, to prevent shock, to minimize the risk of infection, and to get medical help. You should not pull out the object.
> • Press on either side of the object to push together the edges of the wound and control bleeding.
> • Raise the affected area above the level of the heart and help the casualty lie down with his or her legs raised to minimize shock.
> • Build up padding around the object and then bandage over it, taking care not to press on the object.
> • Dial 999 and call an ambulance. Monitor the casualty's vital signs until help arrives.

BLISTERS

A blister is a collection of fluid beneath the outer layer of skin. Most blisters are caused by friction, from badly fitting footwear for example, and are not serious. They usually heal quickly without medical treatment.

WHAT YOU CAN DO

The first thing to do is to remove the source of the friction, by changing footwear, for instance. Whether or not a blister should be deliberately burst is controversial. Most doctors advise against it because of the potential risk of infection but if the blister is tense and painful, the chances are it will burst anyway. Whether the blister has burst naturally or not, you should cover it with a dry, padded, sterile dressing or with a special blister plaster (available from the chemist). These special plasters contain a hydrocolloid gel that cushions the blister and also absorbs any fluid released if the blister breaks. The plasters are designed to be left in place until they come off naturally, by which time the blister will have healed. (The plasters are very sticky, so it's actually quite difficult to remove them early.)

▾ Blisters commonly develop on areas subjected to friction, such as the ball of the foot and heel.

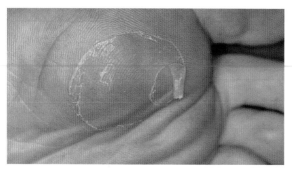

BURNS

Minor burns and scalds are a common occurrence. Follow the advice here on what to do to treat such an injury.

WHAT TO DO

Cool the burn by holding the area under cold running water for ten minutes (time yourself – if you can keep the area under cold water for that length of time it really will help). If there is no running water, any cold liquid will do – even milk. Remove any clothing, watches, or jewellery from the area before it starts to swell. If blisters develop, don't pop them – if you do, you run the risk of infection developing in the burn. Pat the area dry and cover it with a sterile dressing, non-fluffy cloth, or wrap it in cling film. Seek medical advice, if necessary (see box below for guidance).

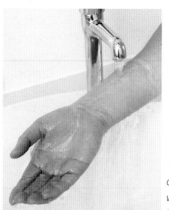

◀ A burn should be cooled in cold running water to stop the burning process.

! SEEK MEDICAL ADVICE NOW

A doctor must see all but the smallest burns on an adult and must check all burns on a child. Take the casualty to the nearest accident and emergency department.
- For a severe burn, start the cooling process and call an ambulance.
- Burns usually need special dressings. Don't be lulled into a false sense of security just because a burn doesn't hurt – no pain can be a sign that the burn is deep and the nerve endings responsible for the sensation of pain have been damaged.

BRUISES

Bruising occurs when blood seeps under the skin following an injury.

WHAT YOU CAN DO

Put an icepack on the affected area as soon as possible. Leave it in place for at least five minutes and reapply it as often as is feasible for up to 72 hours after the injury. If you haven't got an icepack, wrap a bag of frozen peas in a towel – it is just as effective.

Many of my patients also recommend applying arnica cream as a natural remedy to minimize the effects of bruising – scientific studies have failed to show that it works but it may well be worth a try. However, do not use arnica if the skin is broken.

BLACK EYE

A black eye is bruising around the eye. Most are not serious and can be treated with icepacks (as described above) and, if they are sore, paracetamol to relieve the pain. If both eyes are bruised, there could be an underlying fracture of the base of the skull and so a double black eye should always be checked out by a doctor. Also, check the white of the eye – bleeding within the eye (called a hyphaema) could indicate damage to the cornea and should be examined by a doctor.

▾ *Most bruises can be treated by applying an icepack.*

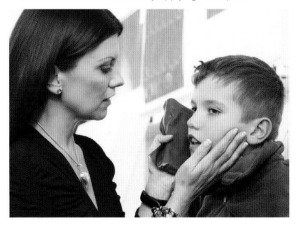

BITES AND STINGS

These are generally more uncomfortable than serious.

INSECT BITES AND STINGS

Put an icepack on the affected area and leave it there for up to ten minutes. Some people are allergic to bites or stings and if the surrounding skin starts to swell, or looks like nettle rash, give them the recommended dose of antihistamines.

If the person has been stung by a bee or wasp and there is a visible sting at the site, brush the sting off with your fingernail or a credit card. Don't use tweezers as you could push more of the poison into the site. Then apply an icepack and cover the area with antihistamine cream. One per cent hydrocortisone cream (available from your chemist) will also help with any itching.

JELLYFISH STINGS

Like most things, prevention is better than cure here – always take local advice and avoid swimming in high-risk areas. Wearing a wetsuit will offer some protection.

If you are stung by a jellyfish, rinse the area immediately with salt water. Don't use fresh water – it may aggravate the sting. Remove any tentacles that remain but be careful not to get stung; you can remove tentacles safely by dusting them with flour and scrape them off with the back of a blunt knife. Vinegar will soothe the site and, as revolting as it may sound, I am reliably assured that if you have no vinegar then urine also works.

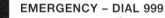

! EMERGENCY – DIAL 999

If the casualty's lips or tongue start to swell, this is a sign of severe allergic reaction – anaphylactic shock – which is a medical emergency. Call an ambulance or take the casualty to accident and emergency immediately.

POISONING

Most poisoning is accidental – children who have drunk a household cleaning fluid or consumed pills thinking they were sweets. In most cases, the taste is enough to prevent children from taking too much and, thankfully, accidental poisoning doesn't usually result in significant problems but it should always be taken seriously.

WHAT YOU CAN DO

If you suspect poisoning, make a note of the time, what you think has been taken (keep any containers or packets), and how much. If the individual is well, phone your local accident and emergency department for advice. But if the person is ill or if you have any doubt about what has been taken, follow the advice in the emergency box below.

WHAT MIGHT THE DOCTOR DO?

The treatment will depend on what has been taken – sometimes the person will be given medicines to make him or her vomit, but if what has been taken is corrosive or caustic, treatment will be aimed at neutralizing the substance.

> **! EMERGENCY – DIAL 999**
>
> If you have any doubt about what the person has taken, or if he or she has swallowed a corrosive or caustic poison, such as bleach, call an ambulance, or go straight to the accident and emergency department. Take any packets or bottles with you to help the medical team identify exactly what is involved.
> • Don't give the person anything to make him or her vomit as a corrosive poison can burn on the way down and again on the way back up.

MUSCLE SPRAINS AND STRAINS

Sprains and strains are common injuries and can be so painful that people often think they have broken a bone, and the person may need an X-ray to diagnose the injury.

WHAT YOU CAN DO

Resting a sprain is essential to allow healing. Icepacks will also help and ideally should be applied for 15 minutes several times a day for three days. A firm bandage will support the sprain, and raising the limb above the level of the heart for as long as possible each day will help to reduce the swelling.

After this initial first aid treatment, the casualty should be encouraged to move the injured area as soon as possible – but gently to begin with. A severe sprain will take up to 12 weeks to heal.

▼ *Applying an icepack and raising the sprained area will help to minimize swelling, bruising, and pain.*

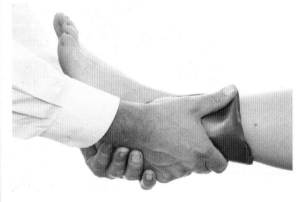

> **! EMERGENCY – DIAL 999**
>
> If you suspect the injury might be a fracture, call an ambulance or take the casualty to the nearest accident and emergency department.

BROKEN BONES

If a limb is very painful to move after an injury, a bone may be broken. If you suspect a broken bone, you must go to the nearest accident and emergency department. An X-ray can confirm whether or not the injury is a fracture.

WHAT YOU CAN DO

Try to keep the injured area as still as possible and immobilize it with a splint – a rolled-up magazine bandaged to the site works well as a temporary splint. The casualty should not have anything to eat or drink until he or she has seen the doctor. In some cases, the bone ends will have moved and need to be manipulated back into position, or even pinned under general anaesthetic, before the limb can be put in plaster. Surgery would have to be delayed if the casualty had consumed food or drink.

▼ *Bandaging a rolled-up magazine around the fracture site will keep it immobilized until the casualty gets medical help.*

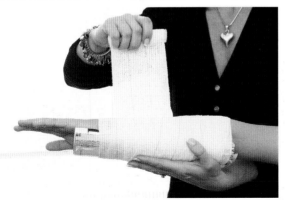

> **! EMERGENCY – DIAL 999**
>
> Call an ambulance if you have no one to support the casualty in the car, or if he or she is in great pain or has to be transported lying down.

HEAD INJURY

These are injuries you need to watch very carefully. Most are just a small bump on the head and there is no other sign of injury. However, a more significnt head injury may have a serious delayed reaction a few days later.

WHAT YOU SHOULD DO

Sit the casualty down, or help him or her to lie down. Give the casualty an icepack to hold against the injured area. If he or she is dazed, has a headache, feels dizzy, cannot remember what happened, or is "knocked out" briefly (no more than 20–30 seconds) but recovers completely, he or she may have concussion and should see a doctor.

COMPRESSION INJURY

Occasionally, there can be bleeding within the skull after a head injury, which eventually starts to press on the brain – compression. The person may be unaffected by the head injury at first but a few hours or days afterwards may begin to deteriorate. He or she may be disorientated, drowsy or confused, have a very bad headache, or weakness – even paralysis – down one side, and may lose consciousness. This is very serious and the person needs urgent medical help.

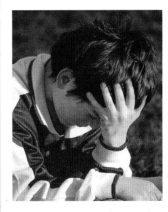

◄ *Most head injuries are minor but all need to be watched carefully in case there is a serious delayed reaction.*

> **! EMERGENCY – DIAL 999**
>
> Call an ambulance if a person starts to show signs of compression injury or loses consciousness hours or days after a head injury.

UNCONSCIOUSNESS

When a person collapses, you need to do three things: make sure the air passages to his or her lungs are clear so that oxygen can enter the body; breathe for him or her, if necessary, to get oxygen into the blood; and keep the blood circulation going so that the blood can take oxygen around the body. This is called cardiopulmonary resuscitation (CPR).

1 Check consciousness – tap the person's shoulder and call out the name; no response means the person is unconscious. Tilt the head back to open the airways. Check breathing – place your cheek by the person's mouth; look along the chest; listen and feel for air from the mouth and nose. If you can't feel anything, the person is not breathing. Get someone to call an ambulance. Ask for a defibrillator (which may be able to restart the heart).

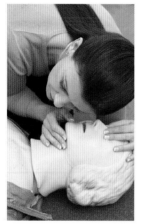

2 Prepare to start chest compressions by finding the place to press down on the chest. Find one of the lowermost ribs using the first two fingers of the hand closest to the person's legs. Slide your fingers along the rib to the point where the lowermost ribs meet the breastbone. Place your middle finger here and your index finger above it on the lower breastbone. Put the heel of your other hand on the breastbone and slide it down until it reaches your index finger. This is where you should press to give chest compressions.

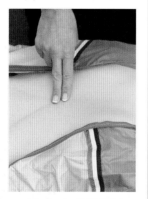

3 Start chest compressions. Place one hand on the centre of the person's chest. Cover this with your other hand. Leaning right over the person's chest with your arms vertical and straight, press down on the chest. Then release the pressure but don't remove your hands – this is a chest compression. Repeat this 30 times at a rate of 100 compressions per minute.

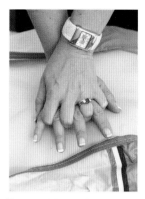

4 Then move to the person's head. Tilt the head back, lift the chin with one hand – this should open the mouth. Pinch the nose closed, then take a breath, place your mouth over the person's mouth, and blow until you see the chest rise. Repeat this. Continue giving 30 chest compressions followed by two breaths of mouth-to-mouth (also known as rescue breaths) until the person starts to breathe or until the ambulance arrives.

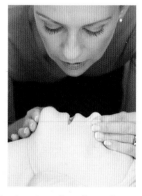

5 If the person is unconscious but breathing, place him or her in the recovery position (see box right), which keeps the airways open.

IF YOU ARE ON YOUR OWN

Give chest compressions and rescue breaths for one minute then call an ambulance. Then resume giving chest compressions and rescue breaths until the ambulance arrives.

CHILDREN AND BABIES

If an unconscious child (one year to puberty) isn't breathing, start by giving the child five rescue breaths, then give 30 chest compressions, but only using one hand, followed by two rescue breaths.

For babies (under 12 months) do the same as for children, but put your mouth over the baby's mouth and nose and only use two fingers for chest compressions.

DR DAWN'S HEALTH CHECK
The recovery position

If you put an unconscious breathing person in this position, it will keep the airways to his or her lungs open and clear. It stops the tongue falling back and blocking the top of the airway and, as the head is lower than the body, fluids can drain from the mouth. It also supports them in a secure position – the back is straight, and the upper arm and leg prevent him or her from rolling forward. You can safely leave a person in this position for a short time – to call for help, for example.

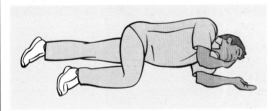

• Kneel beside the person level with his or her chest.
• Place the arm nearest you at right angles to the body and bend it so the forearm is parallel with the body.
• Bring the other arm across the casualty's chest and place his or her palm outwards against the face. Support the leg furthest from you at the knee and pull it up so that the foot is still on the ground.
• Support the casualty's hand against his or her cheek and pull the bent leg towards you, rolling the casualty on to his or her side.
• Bend the upper leg so that it is at a right angle to the body, this prevents them from rolling forwards.
• Adjust the head to make sure the airway is still open and ensure the hand is still under the cheek, supporting the head.

EPILEPTIC SEIZURE

Epilepsy is a condition in which electrical disturbances in the brain cause seizures, or fits. People who suffer from epileptic seizures often carry a card or wear a bracelet indicating this. The seizures can be minor, in which case the person may just appear dazed for a short time. Alternatively, seizures can be major, in which case they generally follow a pattern.

PATTERN OF A MAJOR EPILEPTIC SEIZURE

• Sudden unconsciousness, with the person sometimes letting out a cry.
• The person becomes rigid and arches his or her back.
• Breathing may stop and the person may look "bluish", especially around the lips and nose.
• Convulsive movements begin and the jaw may be clenched. This generally lasts up to five minutes.
• Muscles relax, the person recovers consciousness, then often falls deeply asleep.

WHAT YOU CAN DO

If a person who you know suffers from epileptic seizures suddenly loses consciousness, try to ease the fall. Make a space around them, removing any potentially dangerous objects that he or she could bump into. Protect his or her head, if possible. When the seizure stops, make sure they are is breathing, then place him or her in the recovery position (see box left) until they wake up.

! SEEK MEDICAL ADVICE NOW
If any of the following apply (call an ambulance if necessary):

• The person is unconscious for longer than ten minutes.
• Seizures continue for longer than five minutes.
• The person is having a first seizure, or repeated seizures.

Useful contacts

GENERAL INFORMATION

BBC Online Health
Website: www.bbc.co.uk/health

British Medical Association
BMA House
Tavistock Square
London WC1H 9JP
Tel: 020 7387 4499
Website: www.bma.org.uk

Department of Health
Richmond House
79 Whitehall
London SW1A 2NS
Tel: 020 7210 4850
Website: www.dh.gov.uk

NHS Direct online
Website: www.nhsdirect.nhs.uk

AGEING

Age Concern England
Astral House
1268 London Road
London SW16 4ER
Tel: 020 8765 7200
Website: www.ace.org.uk

Help the Aged (England)
207–221 Pentonville Road
London N1 9UZ
Tel: 020 7278 1114
Website: www.helptheaged.org.uk

ALCOHOL-RELATED PROBLEMS

Addiction Recovery Foundation
193 Victoria Street
London SW1E 5NE
Tel: 020 7233 5333
Website: www.addictiontoday.co.uk

Al-Anon Family Groups UK & Eire
61 Great Dover Street
London SE1 4YF
Helpline: 0845 769 7555
Tel: 020 7403 0888
Website: www.al-anonuk.org.uk

Alcohol Concern
First floor, 8 Shelton Street
London WC2H 9JR
Tel: 020 7395 4000
Website: www.alcoholconcern.org.uk

Alcoholics Anonymous
PO Box 1
Stonebow House
Stonebow
York Y01 7NJ
Helpline: 0845 769 7555
Tel: 01904 644026
Website: www.alcoholics-anonymous.org.uk

ALLERGY AND ASTHMA

Allergy UK
3 White Oak Square
London Road
Swanley
Kent BR8 7AG
Helpline: 01322 619898
Website: www.allergyuk.org

Asthma UK
Summit House
70 Wilson Street
London EC2A 2DB
Helpline: 08457 010203
Tel: 020 7786 4900
Website: www.asthma.org.uk

ALZHEIMER'S DISEASE

Alzheimer's Society
Gordon House
10 Greencoat Place
London SW1P 1PH
Helpline: 0845 300 0336
Tel: 020 7306 0606
Website: www.alzheimers.org.uk

ARTHRITIS

Arthritis Care
18 Stephenson Way
London NW1 2HD
Helpline: 0808 800 4050
Website: www.arthritiscare.org.uk

BACK PAIN

BackCare
16 Elmtree Road
Teddington
Middlesex TW11 8ST
Helpline: 0845 130 2704
Tel: 020 8977 5474
Website: www.backcare.org.uk

BLOOD DISORDERS

Leukaemia CARE
1 Birch Court
Blackpole East
Worcester WR3 8SG
Helpline: 0800 169 6680
Website: www.leukaemiacare.org

Leukaemia Research Fund
43 Great Ormond Street
London WC1N 3JJ
Tel: 020 7405 0101
Website: www.lrf.org.uk

BREAST CANCER

Breakthrough Breast Cancer
246 High Holborn
London WC1V 7EX
Tel: 020 7025 2400
Website: www.breakthrough.org.uk

Breast Cancer Care
Kiln House
210 New Kings Road
London SW6 4NZ
Tel: 020 7384 2984
Website: www.breastcancercare.org.uk

CANCER

Cancer Research UK
PO Box 123
Lincoln's Inn Fields
London WC2A 3PX
Tel: 020 7242 0200
Website: www.cancer.org.uk

Macmillan Cancer Relief
89 Albert Embankment
London SE1 7UQ
Helpline: 0808 808 2020
Website: www.macmillan.org.uk

CHILD ABUSE AND NEGLECT

Childline
45 Folgate Street
London E1 6GL
Helpline: 0800 1111
Tel: 020 7650 3200
Website: www.childline.org.uk

NSPCC
Weston House
42 Curtain Road
London EC2A 3NH
Helpline: 0808 800 5000
Website: www.nspcc.org.uk

COUNSELLING AND PSYCHOTHERAPY

British Association for Counselling and Psychotherapy
BACP House
15 St John's Business Park
Lutterworth
Leicestershire LE17 4HB
Tel: 0870 443 5252
Website: www.bacp.co.uk

RELATE
Tel: 0845 456 1310 or 01788 573241
Website: www.relate.org.uk

DIABETES

Diabetes UK
Macleod House,
10 Parkway
London NW1 7AA
Helpline: 0845 120 2960
Tel: 020 7424 1000
Website: www.diabetes.org.uk

DRUG-RELATED PROBLEMS

National Drugs Helpline
Tel: 0800 776 600
Website: www.talktofrank.com

EAR, NOSE AND THROAT DISORDERS

British Snoring and Sleep Apnoea Association
Castle Court
41 London Road
Reigate RH2 9RJ
Tel: 01737 245638
Website: www.britishsnoring.co.uk

EATING DISORDERS

Beat
103 Prince of Wales Road
Norwich NR1 1DW
Helpline: 0845 634 1414
Website: www.b-eat.co.uk

EPILEPSY
Epilepsy Action
New Anstey House
Gate Way Drive
Yeadon
Leeds LS19 7XY
Helpline: 0808 800 5050
Tel: 0113 210 8800
Website: www.epilepsy.org.uk

National Society for Epilepsy
Chesham Lane
Chalfont St Peter
Bucks SL9 0RJ
Helpline: 01494 601400
Tel: 01494 601300
Website: www.epilepsynse.org.uk

EYE AND VISION DISORDERS
Royal National Institute for the Blind
105 Judd Street
London WC1H 9NE
Helpline: 0845 766 9999
Tel: 020 7388 1266
Website: www.rnib.org.uk

FAMILY PLANNING
Family Planning Association
50 Featherstone Street
London EC1Y 8QU
Helpline: 0845 310 1334
Tel: 020 7608 5240
Website: www.fpa.org.uk

FIRST AID
British Red Cross Society
44 Moorfields
London EC2Y 9AL
Tel: 0870 170 7000
Website: www.redcross.org.uk

St. Andrew's Ambulance Association
St. Andrew's House
48 Milton Street
Glasgow G4 0HR
Tel: 0141 332 4031
Website: www.firstaid.org.uk

St. John Ambulance
27 St John's Lane
London EC1M 4BU
Tel: 0870 010 4950
Website: www.sja.org.uk

HEADACHE
Migraine Trust
The Migraine Trust
55–56 Russell Square
London WC1B 4HP
Tel: 020 7436 1336
Website: www.migrainetrust.org

HEARING DISORDERS
Royal National Institute for Deaf People
19–23 Featherstone Street
London EC1Y 8SL
Helpline: 0808 808 0123
Tel: 020 7296 8000
Website: www.rnid.org.uk

HEART AND CIRCULATION DISORDERS
British Heart Foundation
14 Fitzhardinge Street
London W1H 6DH
Helpline: 0845 070 8070
Tel: 020 7935 0185
Website: www.bhf.org.uk

HIV INFECTION AND AIDS
Terrence Higgins Trust
314–320 Gray's Inn Road
London WC1X 8DP
Helpline: 0845 122 1200
Tel: 020 7812 1600
Website: www.tht.org.uk

IMMUNE DISORDERS
Arthritis Research Campaign
Copeman House
St Mary's Court
St Mary's Gate
Chesterfield
Derbyshire S41 7TD
Tel: 0870 850 5000
Website: www.arc.org.uk

Raynaud's and Scleroderma Association
112 Crewe Road
Alsager
Cheshire ST7 2JA
Tel: 01270 872776
Website: www.raynauds.org.uk

INCONTINENCE
The Continence Foundation
307 Hatton Square
16 Baldwins Gardens
London ECIN 7RJ
Helpline: 0845 345 0165
Tel: 020 7404 6875
Website: www.continence-foundation.org.uk

INFERTILITY
Infertility Network UK
Charter House
43 St Leonards Road
Bexhill-on-Sea TN40 1JA
Helpline: 08701 188088
Tel: 08701 188088
Website: www.infertilitynetworkuk.com

LEARNING DISABILITIES
British Dyslexia Association
98 London Road
Reading RG1 5AU
Helpline: 0118 966 8271
Tel: 0118 966 2677
Website: www.bda-dyslexia.org.uk

LIVER DISORDERS
British Liver Trust
2 Southampton Road
Ringwood BH24 1HY
Tel: 0870 770 8028
Website: www.britishlivertrust.org.uk

LUNG DISORDERS
British Lung Foundaton
73–75 Goswell Road
London EC1V 7ER
Tel: 08458 50 50 20
Website: www.lunguk.org

OSTEOPOROSIS
National Osteoporosis Society
Camerton
Bath BA2 0PJ
Helpline: 0845 450 0230
Website: www.nos.org.uk

PARKINSON'S DISEASE
Parkinson's Disease Society
215 Vauxhall Bridge Road
London SW1V 1EJ
Helpline: 0808 800 0303
Tel: 020 7931 8080
Website: www.parkinsons.org.uk

PREGNANCY AND CHILDBIRTH
Breastfeeding Network
PO Box 11126
Paisley PA2 8YB
Helpline: 0870 900 8787
Website: www.breastfeedingnetwork.org.uk
Miscarriage Association
c/o Clayton Hospital
Northgate
Wakefield
West Yorkshire WF1 3JS
Helpline: 01924 200799
Tel: 01924 200795
Website: www.miscarriageassociation.org.uk

PROSTATE DISORDERS
The Prostate Cancer Charity
3 Angel Walk
London W6 9HX
Helpline: 0800 074 8383
Website: www.prostate-cancer.org.uk

RHEUMATIC DISORDERS
British Society for Rheumatology
Bride House
18–20 Bride Lane
London EC4Y 8EE
Tel: 020 7842 0900
Website: www.rheumatology.org.uk

SEXUAL HEALTH
**British Association for Sexual
and Relationship Therapy**
PO Box 13686
London SW20 9ZH
Tel: 0208 543 2707
Website: www.basrt.org.uk

London Lesbian and Gay Switchboard
PO Box 7324
London N1 9QS
Helpline: 020 7837 7324
Tel: 020 7837 6768
Website: www.llgs.org.uk

SKIN DISORDERS

British Association of Dermatologists
4 Fitzroy Square
London W1T 5HQ
Tel: 0207 383 0266
Website: www.bad.org.uk

National Eczema Society
Hill House
Highgate Hill
London N19 5NA
Helpline: 0870 241 3604
Tel: 020 7281 3553
Website: www.eczema.org

Psoriasis Association
Milton House
7 Milton Street
Northampton NN2 7JG
Tel: 0845 676 0076
Website: www.psoriasis-association.org.uk

Skin Cancer Foundation (US)
Website: www.skincancer.org

Skin Care Campaign
Website: www.skincarecampaign.org

SMOKING

Action on Smoking and Health
102 Clifton Street
London EC2A 4HW
Tel: 020 7739 5902
Website: www.ash.org.uk

SPEECH AND LANGUAGE DISORDERS

The British Stammering Association
15 Old Ford Road
London E2 9PJ
Helpline: 0845 603 2001
Tel: 020 8983 1003
Website: www.stammering.org

STROKE

The Stroke Association
240 City Road
London EC1V 2PR
Helpline: 0845 303 3100
Tel: 020 7566 0300
Website: www.stroke.org.uk

TRAVEL HEALTH

Department of Health
Richmond House
79 Whitehall
London SW1A 2NS
Tel: 020 7210 4850
Website: www.dh.gov.uk

URINARY SYSTEM DISORDERS

British Kidney Patient Association
BKPA
Bordon
Hants GU35 9JZ
Tel: 01420 472021/2
Website: www.britishkidney-pa.co.uk

Cystitis and Overactive Bladder Foundation
76 High Street
Stony Stratford
Buckinghamshire MK11 1AH
Tel: 01908 569169
Website: www.interstitialcystitis.co.uk

WOMEN'S HEALTH

National Association for Premenstrual Syndrome
41 Old Road
East Peckham
Kent TN12 5AP
Helpline: 0870 777 2177
Tel: 0870 777 2178
Website: www.pms.org.uk

National Endometriosis Society
50 Westminster Palace Gardens
Artillery Row
London SW1P 1RR
Helpline: 0808 808 2227
Tel: 020 7222 2781
Website: www.endo.org.uk

INDEX

A

abscesses 39
accidents, first aid 233–41
acne 37, 38
acupressure wristbands 202
addiction
    antidepressants 180–1
    sleeping tablets 196
adenocarcinoma 144
ADHD (attention deficit hyperactivity disorder) 223
adrenaline 178
aerobic exercise 54
ageing
    bones 114
    memory loss 187–8
agnus castus 141, 148
AIDS 171
air travel 201
    deep-vein thrombosis (DVT) 205
    diabetes and 103
    jetlag 205
    travel sickness 202
airway, emergencies 233
alcohol
    and insomnia 196, 197
    and the liver 77–9, 80
    and sex 166
    units 77
alginates 85
allergies
    allergic contact dermatitis 35
    allergic rhinitis 68–9
    asthma 65
    food allergy and intolerance 92–3
    hayfever 68–9
    prickly heat 203
    and snoring 195
alopecia areata 28
alveoli 62, 64
Alzheimer's disease 187, 188–9
anaemia 61
anaphylactic shock 237
angina 51, 52
ankles, swollen 134–5
anorexia nervosa 186, 187
antacids 85
antibiotics
    alcohol and 79
    for ear infections 212
    traveller's diarrhoea 203
antidepressants 149, 180–1
antiperspirants, and breast cancer 152
anus 82

itching 88
    piles (haemorrhoids) 88
apnoea, sleep 195
appendicitis 219
armpits, body odour 40
arms
    carpal tunnel syndrome 126
    repetitive strain injury (RSI) 126
arteries 44
    angina 51, 52
    coronary heart disease (CHD) 50, 52–3
arthritis 118–19
asthma 65
atheroma 52
atherosclerosis 52
athlete's foot 131
atopic eczema 35
autoimmune diseases 118–19
autonomic nervous system 178
avian flu 67

B

babies
    immunizations 225–6
    infantile colic 217
    nappy rash 214, 215
    sticky eye 210
    teething 214
    unconsciousness 241
"baby blues" 182
back pain 120–1
bacteria
    MRSA 125
    probiotics 89
bad breath 21
balanitis 159
baldness 27, 31
basal cell cancer 42
bedwetting 222
bee stings 237
benign coital headache 166
benign prostatic hypertrophy (BPH) 159–60
Bifidobacterium 89
bile 76, 80
bilharzia 111
binge drinking 77
biopsy, breast 150, 152
bird flu 67
bites 237
black cohosh 148
black eye 237
blackheads 38
bladder 104
    cancer 111
    cystitis 107

incontinence 108–10
    and kidney infections 110
bleeding
    after intercourse 139
    first aid 235
    nosebleeds 19
    periods 136, 138–40
    piles (haemorrhoids) 88
    spotting between periods 139
blinking 12, 17
blisters 236
blood
    anaemia 61
    blood clots 74, 60, 190, 205
    cholesterol levels 47–8
    circulation 44
    kidneys and 106
    red blood cells 112
    in semen 157
    see also bleeding
blood pressure 49–50
    and coronary heart disease 53
    kidneys and 106
    and strokes 190
blood sugar levels, diabetes 101–3
blood vessels
    Raynaud's disease 127
    stroke 189–90
    see also arteries; veins
body hair 26
body mass index (BMI) 94
body odour 40
body piercing 43
body temperature
    fevers 209
    hot flushes 147, 148
    taking a temperature 233
boils 39
bones 112, 114
    broken bones 239
    feet 128, 130
    hands 122
    marrow 112, 114
    osteoporosis 116–17, 168
bowels 8
    appendicitis 219
    cancer 97
    constipation 87, 90, 218
    diarrhoea 89, 90, 202–3, 217
    hernias 91
    irritable bowel syndrome (IBS) 90
    potty training 221
    wind 86
brain 174, 176
    Alzheimer's disease 187, 188–9
    children's 206
    depression 180–1
    EEGs (electroencephalogram) 194

PHOTOGRAPHIC CREDITS

The publisher would like to thank the following for their kind permission to reproduce their photographs:

8 Octopus Publishing Group Ltd/Ruth Jenkins; 11 Corbis/John Henley; 15 left Science Photo Library/Sue Ford; 15 right Science Photo Library/Dr P Marazzi; 16 Octopus Publishing Group Ltd/Ruth Jenkins; 17 Science Photo Library/ Custom Medical Stock Photo; 18-19 Octopus Publishing Group Ltd/Ruth Jenkins; 20 Science Photo Library/Dr P Marazzi; 21 Corbis/Royalty-Free; 22 Octopus Publishing Group Ltd/Ruth Jenkins; 23 top Getty Images/Patrick Molnar; 23 bottom Alamy/eStock Photo; 28 left Alamy/Profimedia International s.r.o; 28 right Science Photo Library; 29 Getty Images/ Vincent Besnault; 30 Getty Images/Diana Healey; 35 left Mediscan; 36 left Science Photo Library/Paul Whitehill; 36 right Science Photo Library/Dr P Marazzi; 37 top Science Photo Library/BSIP/Laurent; 37 bottom Science Photo Library/Dr P Marazzi; 39 left Science Photo Library/Dr P Marazzi; 39 right Oxford Scientific Films/BSIP/Chassenet; 40 Alamy/Photick - Image and Click; 41 left Corbis/Norbert Schaefer; 42 top left and right Science Photo Library/Dr P Marazzi; 42 bottom left Science Photo Library/James Stevenson; 43 Science Photo Library/Custom Medical Stock Photo; 47 Octopus Publishing Group Ltd./William Reavell; 49 Octopus Publishing Group Ltd/Ruth Jenkins; 50 Alamy/Maximilian Weinzierl; 51 Octopus Publishing Group Ltd/Ruth Jenkins; 52 Corbis/Royalty-Free; 53-54 Octopus Publishing Group Ltd/Ruth Jenkins; 55 top right Corbis/Jim Cummins; 55 bottom left Alamy/Helene Rogers; 56-57 Octopus Publishing Group Ltd/Ruth Jenkins; 58 Alamy/Tetra Images; 59 Octopus Publishing Group Ltd/Ruth Jenkins; 60 Science Photo Library/BSIP/Mendil; 65 Science Photo Library/Paul Whitehill; 66 Octopus Publishing Group Ltd./William Lingwood; 67 Octopus Publishing Group Ltd/Ruth Jenkins; 68 Science Photo Library/Dr Jeremy Burgess; 69 Getty Images/Suzanne & Nick Geary; 71 Alamy/Photofusion Picture Library; 73 Octopus Publishing Group Ltd/Ruth Jenkins; 78 Octopus Publishing Group Ltd/ Ruth Jenkins; 80 Science Photo Library/Camal, ISM; 81 Octopus Publishing Group Ltd/Ruth Jenkins; 85 Alamy/Image Source; 86 Octopus Publishing Group Ltd./Stephen Conroy; 87 Octopus Publishing Group Ltd./William Lingwood; 88 Photodisc; 90 Science Photo Library/AJ Photo; 92 Octopus Publishing Group Ltd./Ian Wallace; 93 Science Photo Library/James King-Holmes; 94 Octopus Publishing Group Ltd/Ruth Jenkins; 95 Corbis/Fabio Cardoso/zefa; 97 Octopus Publishing Group Ltd/Ruth Jenkins; 100 Science Photo Library/David Hay Jones; 102 Science Photo Library/Ian Boddy; 107 Science Photo Library/BSIP, Bussy/Le Heutre; 109 Octopus Publishing Group Ltd/Ruth Jenkins; 110 Science Photo Library/Adam Gault; 111 Science Photo Library/Zephyr; 115 left Science Photo Library/BSIP,

LA/Filin.Herrera; 115 right Octopus Publishing Group Ltd./Gareth Sambidge; 116 top right Photodisc; 116 bottom left Alamy/Nucleus Medical Art, Inc.; 117 top Corbis/Royalty-Free; 117 bottom Corbis/c Stefan Schuetz/zefa; 118 left Science Photo Library/Zephyr; 118 right Science Photo Library/Dr P Marazzi; 119 Octopus Publishing Group Ltd./Neil Mersh; 120 Science Photo Library/ Ouellette & Theroux, Publiphoto Diffusion; 125 left Alamy/The National Trust Photolibrary; 125 right Getty Images/ Jens & Angelik Buttner; 126 Science Photo Library/Lawrence Lawry; 127 left Corbis/Royalty Free; 127 right Science Photo Library/Dr P Marazzi; 131 left Science Photo Library/Jane Shemilt; 132 Science Photo Library/Dr P Marazzi; 133 Getty Images/Christopher Thomas; 134 Alamy/Medical-on-Line; 135 Science Photo Library/AJ Photo; 139 Science Photo Library/Cristina Pedrazzini; 140 Andrew Lawson Photography; 142-143 Octopus Publishing Group Ltd/Ruth Jenkins; 147 Alamy/mediacolor's; 148 Octopus Publishing Group Ltd./Peter Myers; 149 Digital Vision; 150 Alamy/Chris Rout; 151 Alamy/ImageState; 153 Science Photo Library/Alexander Tsiaras; 157 Science Photo Library/Andrew Syred; 158 Corbis/Grace/zefa; 161 Corbis/Kevin Dodge; 165 Corbis/LWA-Dann Tardif/zefa; 166 Alamy/Everynight Images; 167 left Octopus Publishing Group Ltd/Ruth Jenkins; 167 right Science Photo Library/Ian Hooton; 168 Octopus Publishing Group Ltd/Ruth Jenkins; 169 Getty Images/Jasper James; 171 Science Photo Library/ Dr Klaus Boller; 172 Octopus Publishing Group Ltd/Ruth Jenkins; 173 Science Photo Library/Francis Leroy, Biocosmos; 177 Alamy/Bob Pardue; 178 Alamy/Bildagentur-online; 179 top Image Source; 179 bottom Octopus Publishing Group Ltd./Russell Sadur; 180 Getty Images/Zigy Kaluzny; 181 Photodisc; 182 Science Photo Library/ Chris Knapton; 183 Science Photo Library/BSIP/Laurent; 184 left Octopus Publishing Group Ltd./Stephen Conroy; 184 right Science Photo Library/Coneyl Jay; 185 Andrew Lawson Photography; 186 Science Photo Library/Oscar Burriel; 187 Alamy/Simon Belcher; 188 Octopus Publishing Group Ltd./William Reavell; 189 Getty Images/Justin Pumfrey; 190 Science Photo Library/Zephyr; 191 Science Photo Library/Catherine Pouedras/Eurelios; 195 Corbis/Royalty-Free; 196 Getty Images/Mark Douet; 201 Octopus Publishing Group Ltd/Ruth Jenkins; 202 left Sea-Band; 202 right Alamy/ImageState; 203 Science Photo Library/Logical Images; 204 Alamy/Chris A Crumley; 205 Science Photo Library/Samuel Ashfield; 209 top BananaStock; 209 bottom Science Photo Library/Dr H C Robinson; 210 Science Photo Library/Dr P Marazzi; 210 left Science Photo Library/Simon Fraser; 211 right Octopus Publishing Group Ltd/Ruth Jenkins; 213 Science Photo Library/Michael Donne; 214 left BananaStock; 214 bottom right Science Photo Library/Dr P Marazzi; 215 top right Science Photo Library/Dr P Marazzi; 215 bottom left Alamy/Bubbles Photolibrary; 216 Mediscan; 218 Alamy/Picture Partners; 219 BananaStock; 220 Getty Images/Pascal Rondeau; 221 left Science Photo Library/Oscar Burriel; 221 right BananaStock; 222 Alamy/Christa Stadtler; 223 Science Photo Library/BSIP/ Mendil; 224 Alamy/Bubbles Photolibrary; 227 top left Science Photo Library/Ian Boddy; 227 bottom right Alamy/Tim Caddick; 228 left Science Photo Library/Lowell Georgia; 228 right Alamy/Sally and Richard Greenhill; 229 left Science Photo Library/Dr P Marazzi; 229 right Wellcome Photo Library; 232-235 Octopus Publishing Group Ltd/Ruth Jenkins; 236 left Alamy/Ian Leonard; 236 right-239 left Octopus Publishing Group Ltd/Ruth Jenkins; 239 right Science Photo Library/Mark Clarke; 240 Octopus Publishing Group Ltd/Ruth Jenkins

AUTHOR ACKNOWLEDGMENTS

I would like to thank all the friends, colleagues and patients that have helped to make this book possible. There are so many of you, that I can't hope to mention you all by name, but there are a few really important people without whom this book simply wouldn't have happened.

My special thanks go to my agent Debbie Catchpole at Fresh Partners for encouraging me to put pen to paper, to David Lamb at Mitchell-Beazley for believing in me, to the editorial team, Hannah Barnes-Murphy, Hannah McEwen, the late Daphne Razazan and Jemima Dunne for their unerring support, and of course to my husband Graham for being my rock.

Last but not least, I would like to thank Moreen Niblett, Rachel Hinds and Shelly Owens who cleaned my home, mucked out my horses and ferried my children while I locked myself in the office – without you, I would still be on the first chapter!